Virtual Clinical Excursions—Medical-Surgical

for

Black and Hawks
Medical-Surgical Nursing:
Clinical Management for Positive Outcomes, 7th Edition

Virtual Clinical Excursions—Medical-Surgical

for

Black and Hawks
Medical-Surgical Nursing:
Clinical Management for Positive Outcomes, 7th Edition

prepared by

Dorothy Mathers, RN, MSN
Associate Professor, Nursing
Pennsylvania College of Technology
Williamsport, Pennsylvania

software developed by

Wolfsong Informatics, LLC
Tucson, Arizona

ELSEVIER
SAUNDERS

ELSEVIER
SAUNDERS

1600 John F. Kennedy Boulevard
Suite 1800
Philadelphia, Pennsylvania 19103-2899

VIRTUAL CLINICAL EXCURSIONS — MEDICAL-SURGICAL FOR   ISBN 1-4160-0102-6
BLACK AND HAWKS: MEDICAL-SURGICAL NURSING:
CLINICAL MANAGEMENT FOR POSITIVE OUTCOMES,
SEVENTH EDITION
Copyright © 2006, Elsevier Inc.

Notice

Knowledge and best practice in this field are constantly changing. As new research and experience broaden our knowledge, changes in practice, treatment and drug therapy may become necessary or appropriate. Readers are advised to check the most current information provided (i) on procedures featured or (ii) by the manufacturer of each product to be administered, to verify the recommended dose or formula, the method and duration of administration, and contraindications. It is the responsibility of the practitioner, relying on their own experience and knowledge of the patient, to make diagnoses, to determine dosages and the best treatment for each individual patient, and to take all appropriate safety precautions. To the fullest extent of the law, neither the Publisher nor the Authors assumes any liability for any injury and/or damage to persons or property arising out or related to any use of the material contained in this book.

International Standard Book Number 1-4160-0102-6

Senior Editor, Nursing: *Tom Wilhelm*
Managing Editor: *Jeff Downing*
Associate Developmental Editor: *Jennifer Anderson*
Project Manager: *Joy Moore*

Printed in the United States of America

Last digit is the print number: 9   8   7   6   5   4   3   2   1

*Workbook
prepared by*

Dorothy Mathers, RN, MSN
Associate Professor, Nursing
Pennsylvania College of Technology
Williamsport, Pennsylvania

Textbook

Joyce M. Black, PhD, CPSN, CCCN, CWCN
Assistant Professor
College of Nursing
University of Nebraska Medical Center
Omaha, Nebraska

Jane Hokanson Hawks, DNSc, RN, BC
Associate Professor of Nursing
Midland Lutheran College
Fremont, Nebraska

Reviewers

Gina Long, RN, DNSc

Assistant Professor
Department of Nursing
College of Health Professions
Northern Arizona University
Flagstaff, Arizona

Diana Mixon, BSN, MSN

Associate Professor
Department of Nursing
Boise State University
Boise, Idaho

Contents

Unit 9—Circulatory Disorders

Unit 10—Oxygenation Disorders

Unit 11—Sensory Disorders

Unit 12—Cognitive and Perceptual Disorders

Unit 13—Protective Disorders

Table of Contents
Black and Hawks
Medical-Surgical Nursing:
Clinical Management for Positive Outcomes, 7th Edition

Getting Started

GETTING SET UP

■ MINIMUM SYSTEM REQUIREMENTS

WINDOWS™

Windows XP, 2000, 98, ME, NT 4.0 (Recommend Windows XP/2000)
Pentium® III processor (or equivalent) @ 600 MHz (Recommend 800 MHz or better)
128 MB of RAM (Recommend 256 MB or more)
800 x 600 screen size (Recommend 1024 x 768)
Thousands of colors
12x CD-ROM drive
Soundblaster 16 soundcard compatibility
Stereo speakers or headphones

Note: Virtual Clinical Excursion—Medical-Surgical for Windows will require a minimal amount of disk space to install icons and required dll files for Windows 98/ME.

MACINTOSH®

MAC OS X (10.2 or higher)
Apple Power PC G3 @ 500 MHz or better
128 MB of RAM (Recommend 256 MB or more)
800 x 600 screen size (Recommend 1024 x 768)
Thousands of colors
12x CD-ROM drive
Stereo speakers or headphones

1

■ INSTALLATION INSTRUCTIONS

WINDOWS

1. Insert the *Virtual Clinical Excursion—Medical-Surgical* CD-ROM.
2. Inserting the CD should automatically bring up the setup screen if the current product is not already installed.
   a. If the setup screen does not appear automatically (and *Virtual Clinical Excursion—Medical-Surgical* has not been installed already), navigate to the "My Computer" icon on your desktop or in your Start menu.
   b. Double-click on your CD-ROM drive.
   c. If installation does not start at this point:
      (1) Click the **Start** icon on the task bar and select the **Run** option.
      (2) Type d:\setup.exe (where "d:\" is your CD-ROM drive) and press **OK**.
      (3) Follow the onscreen instructions for installation.
3. Follow the onscreen instructions during the setup process.

MACINTOSH

1. Insert the *Virtual Clinical Excursion—Medical-Surgical* CD in the CD-ROM drive. The disk icon will appear on your desktop.

2. Double-click on the disk icon.

3. Double-click on the MEDICAL-SURGICAL_MAC run file.

NOTE: *Virtual Clinical Excursion—Medical-Surgical* for Macintosh does not have an installation setup and can only be run directly from the CD.

■ HOW TO USE VIRTUAL CLINICAL EXCURSIONS—MEDICAL-SURGICAL

WINDOWS

1. Double-click on the *Virtual Clinical Excursion—Medical-Surgical* icon located on your desktop.
2. Or navigate to the program via the Windows Start menu.

NOTE: Windows 98/ME will require you to restart your computer before running the *Virtual Clinical Excursion—Medical-Surgical* program.

MACINTOSH

1. Insert the *Virtual Clinical Excursion—Medical-Surgical* CD in the CD-ROM drive. The disk icon will appear on your desktop.

2. Double-click on the disk icon.

3. Double-click on the MEDICAL-SURGICAL_MAC run file.

■ SCREEN SETTINGS

For best results, your computer monitor resolution should be set at a minimum of 800 x 600. The number of colors displayed should be set to "thousands or higher" (High Color or 16 bit) or "millions of colors" (True Color or 24 bit).

Windows™

1. From the **Start** menu, select **Control Panel** (on some systems, you will first go to **Settings**, then to **Control Panel**).
2. Double-click on the **Display** icon.
3. Click on the **Settings** tab.
4. Under **Screen area** use the slider bar to select **800 by 600 pixels**.
5. Access the **Colors** drop-down menu by clicking on the down arrow.
6. Select **High Color (16 bit)** or **True Color (24 bit)**.
7. Click on **OK**.
8. You may be asked to verify the setting changes. Click **Yes**.
9. You may be asked to restart your computer to accept the changes. Click **Yes**.

Macintosh®

1. Select the **Monitors** control panel.
2. Select **800 x 600** (or similar) from the **Resolution** area.
3. Select **Thousands** or **Millions** from the **Color Depth** area.

■ WEB BROWSERS

Supported web browsers include Microsoft Internet Explorer (IE) version 5.0 or higher and Netscape version 4.5 or higher. *Note that Netscape version 6.0 is not supported at this time, although versions 6.2 and higher are supported.*

If you use America Online (AOL) for web access, you will need AOL version 4.0 or higher and IE 5.0 or higher. Do not use earlier versions of AOL with earlier versions of IE, because you will have difficulty accessing many features.

For best results with AOL:
*   Connect to the Internet using AOL version 4.0 or higher.
*   Open a private chat within AOL (this allows the AOL client to remain open, without asking whether you wish to disconnect while minimized).
*   Minimize AOL.
*   Launch a recommended browser.

■ TECHNICAL SUPPORT

Technical support for this product is available between 7:30 a.m. and 7 p.m. CST, Monday through Friday. Before calling, be sure that your computer meets the minimum system requirements to run this software. Inside the United States and Canada, call 1-800-692-9010. Outside North America, call 314-872-8370. You may also fax your questions to 314-997-5080 or contact Technical Support through e-mail: technical.support@elsevier.com.

ACCESSING *Virtual Clinical Excursions—Medical-Surgical* FROM EVOLVE

The product you have purchased is part of the Evolve family of online courses and learning resources. Please read the following information completely to get started.

To access your instructor's course on Evolve:

Your instructor will provide you with the username and password needed to access their specific course on the Evolve Learning System. Once you have received this information, please follow these instructions:

1. Go to the Evolve student page (http://evolve.elsevier.com/student)

2. Enter your username and password in the **Login to My Evolve** area and click the **Login** button.

3. You will be taken to your personalized **My Evolve** page where the course will be listed in the **My Courses** module.

TECHNICAL REQUIREMENTS

To use an Evolve course, you will need access to a computer that is connected to the Internet and equipped with web browser software that supports frames. For optimal performance, it is recommended that you have speakers and use a high-speed Internet connection. However, slower dial-up modems (56 K minimum) are acceptable.

Whichever browser you use, the browser preferences must be set to enable cookies and Java/JavaScript and the cache must be set to reload every time.

<u>**Enable Cookies**</u>

Browser	Steps
Internet Explorer 5.0 or higher	1. Select **Tools**. 2. Select **Internet Options**. 3. Select **Security** tab. 4. Make sure **Internet** (globe) is highlighted. 5. Select **Custom Level** button. 6. Scroll down the **Security Settings** list. 7. Under **Cookies** heading, make sure **Enable** is selected. 8. Click **OK**.
Internet Explorer 6.0	1. Select **Tools**. 2. Select **Internet Options**. 3. Select **Privacy** tab. 4. Use the slider (slide down) to **Accept All Cookies**. 5. Click **OK**. **-OR-** 4. Click the **Advanced** button. 5. Click the check box next to **Override Automatic Cookie Handling**. 6. Click the **Accept** buttons under **First-party Cookies** and **Third-party Cookies**. 7. Click **OK**.
Netscape Communicator or Navigator 4.5 or higher	1. Select **Edit**. 2. Select **Preferences**. 3. Click **Advanced**. 4. Click **Accept all cookies**. 5. Click **OK**.
Netscape Communicator or Navigator 6.1 or higher	1. Select **Edit**. 2. Select **Preferences**. 3. Select **Privacy & Security**. 4. Select **Cookies**. 5. Select **Enable All Cookies**.

Enable Java

Browser	Steps
Internet Explorer 5.0 or higher	1. Select **Tools**. 2. Select **Internet Options**. 3. Select the **Advanced** tab. 4. Locate **Microsoft VM**. 5. Make sure the **Java console enabled** and **Java logging enabled** boxes are checked. 6. Click **OK**. 7. Restart your computer if you checked the **Java console enabled** box.
Netscape Communicator or Navigator 4.5 or higher	1. Select **Edit** 2. Select **Preferences**. 3. Select **Advanced**. 4. Make sure the **Enable Java** and **Enable JavaScript** boxes are checked. 5. Click **OK**.

Set Cache to Always Reload a Page

Browser	Steps
Internet Explorer 5.0 or higher	1. Select **Tools**. 2. Select **Internet Options**. 3. Select the **General** tab. 4. Select **Settings** from within the **Temporary Internet Files** section. 5. Select the **Every visit to the page** button. 6. Click **OK**.
Netscape Communicator or Navigator 4.5 or higher	1. Select **Edit** 2. Select **Preferences**. 2. Click the + or → icon next to the **Advanced** to see more options. 3. Select **Cache**. 4. Select the **Every time** button at the bottom. 5. Click **OK**.

Plug-Ins

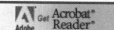 **Adobe Acrobat Reader**—With the free Acrobat Reader software you can view and print Adobe PDF files. Many Evolve products offer student and instructor manuals, checklists, and more in this format!

Download at: http://www.adobe.com

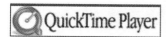 **Apple QuickTime**—Install this to hear word pronunciations, heart and lung sounds, and many other helpful audio clips within Evolve Online Courses!

Download at: http://www.apple.com

 Macromedia Flash Player—This player will enhance your viewing of many Evolve web pages, as well as educational short-form to long-form animation within the Evolve Learning System!

Download at: http://www.macromedia.com

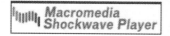 **Macromedia Shockwave Player**—Shockwave is best for viewing the many interactive learning activities within Evolve Online Courses!

Download at: http: //www.macromedia.com

 Microsoft Word Viewer—With this viewer Microsoft Word users can share documents with those who don't have Word, and users without Word can open and view Word documents. Many Evolve products have testbank, student and instructor manuals, and other documents available for downloading and viewing on your own computer!

Download at: *http://www.microsoft.com*

 Microsoft PowerPoint Viewer—View PowerPoint 97, 2000, and 2002 presentations even if you don't have PowerPoint with this viewer. Many Evolve products have slides available for downloading and viewing on your own computer!

Download at: *http://www.microsoft.com*

SUPPORT INFORMATION

Live support is available to customers in the United States and Canada from 7:30 a.m. to 7:00 p.m. (Central Time), Monday through Friday by calling, **1-800-401-9962**. You can also send an email to evolve-support@elsevier.com.

There is also **24/7 support information** available on the Evolve website (http://evolve.elsevier.com), including:

- Guided Tours
- Tutorials
- Frequently Asked Questions (FAQs)
- Online Copies of Course User Guides
- And much more!

A QUICK TOUR

Welcome to *Virtual Clinical Excursions—Medical-Surgical*, a virtual hospital setting in which you can work with multiple complex patient simulations and also learn to access and evaluate the information resources that are essential for high-quality patient care.

The virtual hospital, Pacific View Regional Hospital, has realistic architecture and access to patient rooms, a Nurses' Station, and a Medication Room.

■ BEFORE YOU START

Make sure you have your textbook nearby when you use the *Virtual Clinical Excursions—Medical-Surgical* CD. You will want to consult topic areas in your textbook frequently while working with the CD and using this workbook.

■ HOW TO SIGN IN

- Enter your name on the Student Nurse identification badge.
- Now click the down arrow next to **Select Period of Care**. This drop-down menu gives you four periods of care from which to choose. In Periods of Care 1 through 3, you can actively engage in patient assessment, entry of data in the electronic patient record (EPR), and medication administration. Period of Care 4 presents the day in review. Highlight and click the appropriate period of care. (For this quick tour, choose **Period of Care 2**.)
- Click **Go** in the lower right side of the screen.
- This takes you to the Patient List screen (see example on page 11). Only the patients on the floor you choose (Medical-Surgical) are available. Note that the virtual time is provided in the box at the lower left corner of the screen (1115, since we chose Period of Care 2).

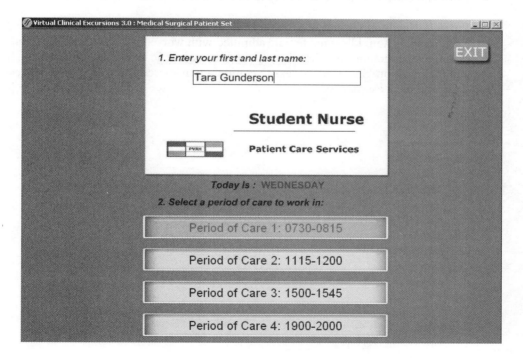

■ **PATIENT LIST**

MEDICAL-SURGICAL UNIT

Harry George (Room 401)
Osteomyelitis—A middle-aged Caucasian male admitted from a homeless shelter with an infected leg. He has complications of type 2 diabetes mellitus, alcohol abuse, nicotine addiction, poor pain control, and complex psychosocial issues.

Jacqueline Catanazaro (Room 402)
Asthma—A middle-aged Caucasian female admitted with an acute asthma exacerbation and suspected pneumonia. She has complications of chronic schizophrenia, noncompliance with medication therapy, obesity, and herniated disc.

Piya Jordan (Room 403)
Bowel obstruction—An older Asian female admitted with a colon mass and suspected adenocarcinoma. She undergoes a right hemicolectomy. This patient's complications include atrial fibrillation, hypokalemia, and symptoms of meperidine toxicity.

Clarence Hughes (Room 404)
Degenerative joint disease—An older African-American male admitted for a left total knee replacement. His preparations for discharge are complicated by the development of a pulmonary embolus and the need for ongoing intravenous therapy.

Pablo Rodriguez (Room 405)
Metastatic lung carcinoma—An older Hispanic male admitted with symptoms of dehydration and malnutrition. He has chronic pain secondary to multiple subcutaneous skin nodules and psychosocial concerns related to family issues with his approaching death.

Patricia Newman (Room 406)
Pneumonia—A middle-aged female admitted with worsening pulmonary function and an acute respiratory infection. Her chronic emphysema is complicated by heavy smoking, hypertension, and malnutrition. She needs access to community resources such as a smoking cessation program and meal assistance.

■ HOW TO SELECT A PATIENT

- You can choose one or more patients to work with from the Patient List by clicking the box to the left of the patient name(s). (In order to receive a scorecard for a patient, the patient must be selected before proceeding to the Nurses' Station.)
- Click on **Get Report** to the right of the medical records number (MRN) to view a summary of the patient's care during the 12-hour period before your arrival on the unit.
- When you are ready to begin your care, click on **Go to Nurses' Station** in the right lower corner.

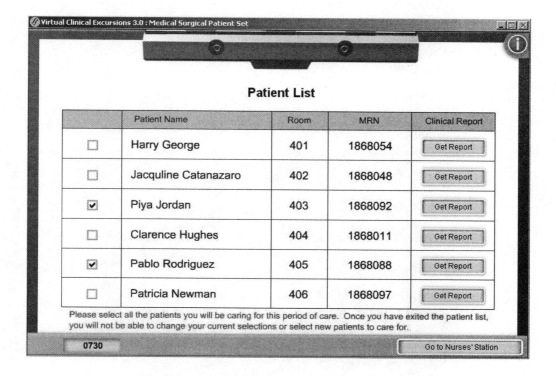

Copyright © 2006 by Elsevier, Inc. All rights reserved.

◼ HOW TO FIND A PATIENT'S RECORDS

NURSES' STATION

Within the Nurses' Station, you will see:

1. A clipboard that contains the patient list for that floor.
2. A chart rack with patient charts labeled by room number, a notebook labeled Kardex, and a notebook labeled MAR (Medication Administration Record).
3. A desktop computer with access to the Electronic Patient Record (EPR).
4. A tool bar across the top of the screen that can also be used to access the Patient List, EPR, Chart, MAR, and Kardex. This tool bar is also accessible from each patient's room.
5. A Drug Guide containing information about the medications you are able to administer to your patients.

As you run your cursor over an item, it will be highlighted. To select, simply double-click on the item. As you use these resources, you will always be able to return to the Nurses' Station by clicking on the **Return to Nurses' Station** bar located in the right lower corner of your screen.

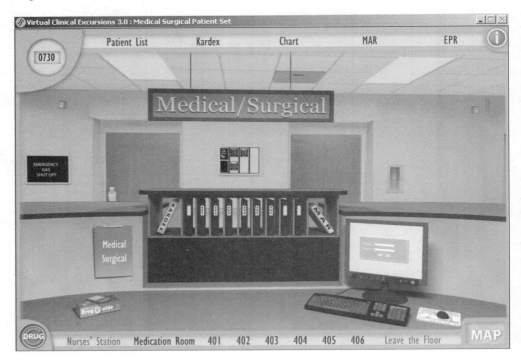

MEDICATION ADMINISTRATION RECORD (MAR)

The MAR icon located in the tool bar at the top of your screen accesses current 24-hour medications for each patient. Click on the icon and the MAR will open. (*Note:* You can also access the MAR by clicking on the blue MAR notebook on the far right side of the book rack in the center of the screen.) Within the MAR, tabs on the right side of the screen allow you to select patients by room number. Be careful to make sure you select the correct tab number for *your* patient rather than simply reading the first record that appears after the MAR opens. Each MAR sheet lists the following:

- Medications
- Route and dosage of medications
- Times of administration of medication

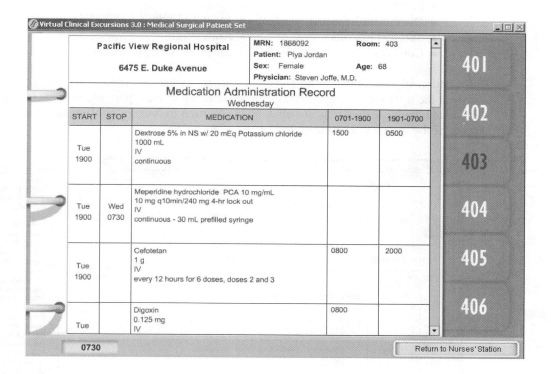

Note: The MAR changes each day. Expired MARs are stored in the patients' charts.

CHARTS

To access patient charts, either click on the **Chart** icon at the top of your screen or anywhere within the chart rack in the center of the Nurses' Station screen. When the close-up view appears, the individual charts are labeled by room number. To open a chart, click on the room number of the patient whose chart you wish to review. The patient's name and allergies will appear, along with a list of tabs on the right side of the screen, allowing you to view the following data:

- Allergies
- Physician's Orders
- Physician's Notes
- Nurse's Notes
- Laboratory Reports
- Diagnostic Reports
- Surgical Reports
- Consultations

- Patient Education
- History and Physical
- Nursing Admission
- Expired MARs
- Consents
- Mental Health
- Admissions
- Emergency Department

Information appears in real time. The entries are in reverse chronological order, so use the down arrow at the right side of the chart page to scroll down to view previous entries. Flip from tab to tab to view multiple data fields or click on the **Return to Nurses' Station** bar in the lower right corner of the screen to exit the chart.

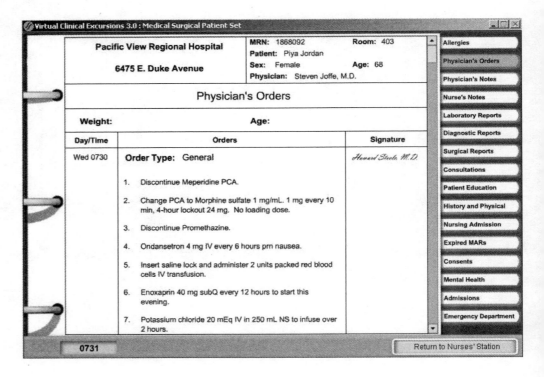

ELECTRONIC PATIENT RECORD (EPR)

The EPR can be accessed from the computer in the Nurses' Station or from the EPR icon located in the tool bar at the top of your screen. To access a patient's EPR:

- Click on either the computer screen or the **EPR** icon.
- Your user name and password are automatically filled in.
- Click on **Login** to enter the EPR.

The EPR used in Pacific View Regional Hospital represents a composite of commercial versions being used in hospitals. You can access the EPR:

- for a patient (by room number).
- to review existing data.
- to enter data you collect while working with a patient.

The EPR is updated daily, so no matter what day or part of a shift you are working, there will be a current EPR with the patient's data from the past days of the current hospital stay. This type of simulated EPR allows you to examine how data for different attributes have changed over time, as well as to examine data for all of a patient's attributes at a particular time. The EPR is fully functional (as it is in a real-life hospital). You can enter such data as blood pressure, breath sounds, and certain treatments. The EPR will not, however, allow you to enter data for a previous time period. Use the arrows at the bottom of the screen to move forward and backward in time.

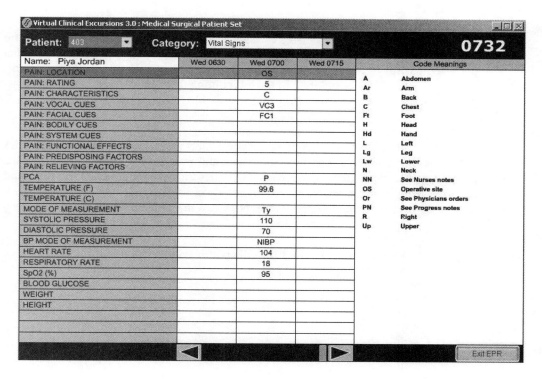

At the top of the EPR screen, you can choose patients by their room numbers. In addition, you have access to 17 different categories of patient data. To change patients or data categories, click the down arrow to the right of the room number or category.

The categories of patient data in the EPR as as follows:

- Vital Signs
- Respiratory
- Cardiovascular
- Neurologic
- Gastrointestinal
- Excretory
- Musculoskeletal
- Integumentary
- Reproductive
- Psychosocial
- Wounds and Drains
- Activity
- Hygiene and Comfort
- Safety
- Nutrition
- IV
- Intake and Output

Remember, each hospital selects its own codes. The codes used in the EPR at Pacific View Regional Hospital may be different from ones you have seen in clinical rotations that have computerized patient records. Take some time to acquaint yourself with the codes. Within the Vital Signs category, click on any item in the left column (e.g., heart rate). In the far-right column, you will see a list of code meanings for the possible findings and/or descriptors for that assessment area.

You will use the codes to record the data you collect as you work with patients. Click on the box in the last time column to the right of the data and wait for the code meanings applicable to that entry to appear. Select the appropriate code to describe your assessment findings and type it in the box. (*Note:* If no cursor appears within the box, click on the box again until the blue shading disappears and the blinking cursor appears.) Once the data are typed in this box, they are entered into the patient's record for this period of care only.

To leave the EPR, click on **Exit EPR** in the bottom right corner of the screen.

■ **VISITING A PATIENT**

From the Nurses' Station, click on the room number of the patient you wish to visit in the tool bar at the bottom of your screen. Once you are inside the room, you will see a still photo of your patient in the top left corner. To verify that this is the patient you have chosen, click on the **Check Armband** icon to the right of the photo. The patient's identification data will appear. If you click on **Check Allergies** (the next icon to the right), a list of the patient's allergies (if any) will replace the photo.

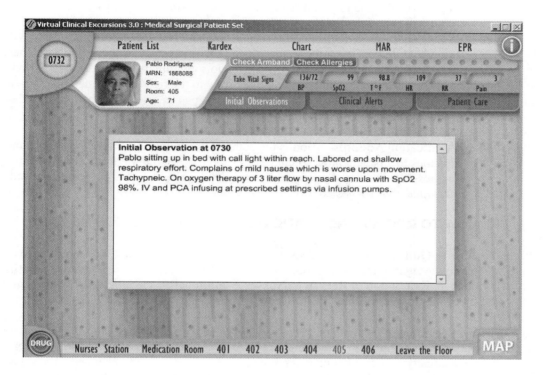

Also located in the patient's room are multiple icons you may use to assess the patient or the patient's medications. A clock is provided in the upper left corner of the room to monitor your progress in real time.

- The tool bar across the top of the screen allows you to check the **Patient List**, access the **EPR** to check or enter data, and view the patient's **Chart**, **MAR**, or **Kardex**.

- The **Take Vital Signs** icon allows you to measure the patient's up-to-the-minute blood pressure, oxygen saturation, temperature, heart rate, respiratory rate, and pain level.

- When you click on **Initial Observations**, a description appears in the text box under the patient's photo, allowing you a "look" at the patient as if you had just stepped in. To the right of this icon is **Clinical Alerts**, a resource that allows you to make decisions about priority medication interventions based on emerging data collected in real time. Check this screen throughout your period of care to avoid missing critical information related to recently ordered or STAT medications.

- Clicking on the **Patient Care** icon opens up three specific learning environments within the patient room: **Physical Assessment**, **Nurse-Client Interactions**, and **Medication Administration**.

- To perform a **Physical Assessment**, choose a body area (such as **Head & Neck**) by clicking on the appropriate icon in the column of yellow buttons. This activates a list of system sub-categories for that body area (e.g., see **Sensory**, **Neurologic**, etc. in the green boxes). After you click on the system that you wish to evaluate, a still photo and text box appear, describing the assessment findings. The still photo is a "snapshot" of how an assessment of this area might be done or what the finding might look like. For every body area, there is also a **Equipment** button located on the far right of the screen.

- To the right of the Physical Assessment icon is **Nurse-Client Interactions**. Clicking on this icon will reveal the times and titles of any videos available for viewing. (*Note:* If the video you wish to see is not listed, this means you have not yet reached the correct virtual time to view that video. Check the virtual clock; you may return to access the video once its designated time has occurred—as long as you do so within the corresponding period of care.) To view a listed video, click on the white arrow to the right of the video title. Use the square control buttons below the video to start, stop, pause, rewind, or fast-forward the action or to mute the sound.

- **Medication Administration** is the pathway that allows you to review and administer medications to a patient after you have prepared them in the Medication Room. This process is addressed further in the *How to Prepare Medications* section (pages 19-20) and in *A Detailed Tour* (pages 26-30).

■ HOW TO QUIT, CHANGE PATIENTS, OR CHANGE PERIOD OF CARE

How to Quit: From most screens, you may click the **Leave the Floor** icon on the bottom tool bar to the right of the patient room numbers. (*Note:* From some screens, you will first need to click an **Exit** button or **Return to Nurses' Station** before clicking **Leave the Floor**.) When the Floor Menu appears, click **Exit** to leave the program.

How to Change Patients or Period of Care: To change patients, simply click on the new patient's room number. (You cannot receive a scorecard for a new patient, however, unless you have already selected that patient on the Patient List screen.) To change to a new period of care or restart the virtual clock for a new patient, click the **Leave the Floor** icon and then **Restart**.

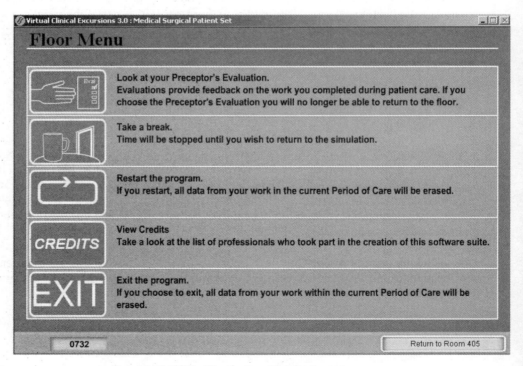

■ HOW TO PREPARE MEDICATIONS

From the Nurses' Station or the patient's room, you can access the Medication Room by clicking on the icon in the tool bar at the bottom of your screen to the left of the patient room numbers.

In the Medication Room you have access to the following (from left to right):

- A preparation area is located on the counter under the cabinets. To begin the medication preparation process, click on the tray on the counter or click on the **Preparation** icon at the top of the screen. The next screen leads you through a preparation sequence (called the Preparation Wizard) to prepare medications one at a time for administration to a patient. However, no medication has been selected at this time. We will do this while working with a patient in *A Detailed Tour*. To exit this screen, click on **View the Medication Room**.

- To the right of the cabinets (and above the refrigerator), IV storage bins are provided. Click on the bins themselves or on the **IV Storage** icon at the top of the screen. The bins are labeled **Microinfusion**, **Small Volume**, and **Large Volume**. Click on an individual bin to see a list of its contents. No medications are available in the bins at this time, but if they were, you could click on an individual medication and its label would appear to the right under the patient's name. Next, you would click **Put Medication on Tray**. If you ever change your mind or choose the incorrect medication, you can reverse your actions by clicking on **Put Medication in Bin**. Click **Close Bin** in the right bottom corner to exit. **View Medication Room** brings you back to a full view of the entire room.

- A refrigerator is located under the IV storage bins to hold any medications that must be stored below room temperature. Click on it to remove your medications; then click **Close Door**. You can also access this area by clicking the **Refrigerator** icon at the top of the screen.

- To prepare controlled substances, click the **Automated System** icon at the top of the screen or click the computer monitor located to the right of the IV storage bins. A login screen will appear; your name and password are automatically filled in. Click **Login**. Select a patient to log medications out for; then select the drawer you wish to open. Click **Open Drawer**, choose **Put Medication on Tray**, and then click **Close Drawer**.

- Next to the Automated System is a set of drawers identified by patient room number. To access these, click on the drawers themselves or on the **Unit Dosage** icon at the top of the screen. This provides a close-up view of the drawers. Click on the room number of the patient you are working with to open that drawer. Next, click on the medication you would like to prepare for the patient, and a label appears to the right under the patient's name, listing strength, units, and dosage per unit. You can **Open** and **Close** this medication label by clicking the appropriate icon. To exit, click **Close Drawer**; then click **View Medication Room**.

At any time, you can learn about a medication you wish to prepare for a patient by clicking on the **Drug** icon in the bottom left corner of the medication room screen or by clicking the **Drug Guide** book on the counter to the right of the unit dosage drawers. The **Drug Guide** provides information about the medications commonly included in nursing drug handbooks. Nutritional supplements and maintenance intravenous fluid preparations are not included.

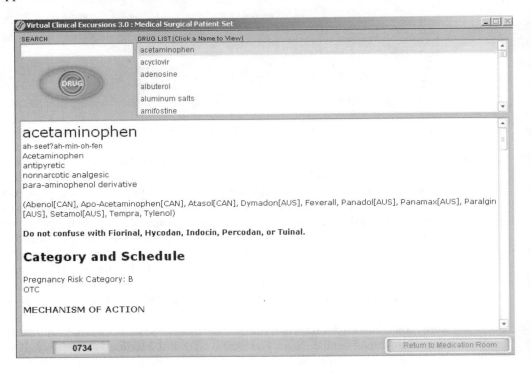

To access the MAR to review the medications ordered for a patient, click on the **MAR** icon located in the tool bar at the top of your screen. You may also click the **Review MAR** icon in the tool bar at the bottom of your screen from inside each medication storage area.

After you have chosen and prepared your medications, return to the patient's room to administer them by clicking on the room number in the bottom tool bar. Once inside the patient's room, click on **Medication Administration** and follow the administration sequence.

■ PRECEPTOR'S EVALUATIONS

When you have finished a session, click on **Leave the Floor** to go to the Floor Menu. At this point, you can click on the icon next to **Look at your Preceptor's Evaluation** to receive a scorecard that provides feedback on the work you completed during patient care.

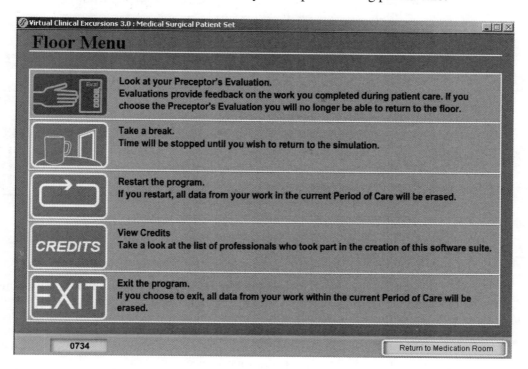

Evaluations are available for each patient you signed in for. Click on any of the **Medication Scorecard** icons to see an example. The scorecard compares the medications you administered to a patient during a period of care with what should have been administered. Table A lists the correct medications. Table B lists any medications that were administered incorrectly.

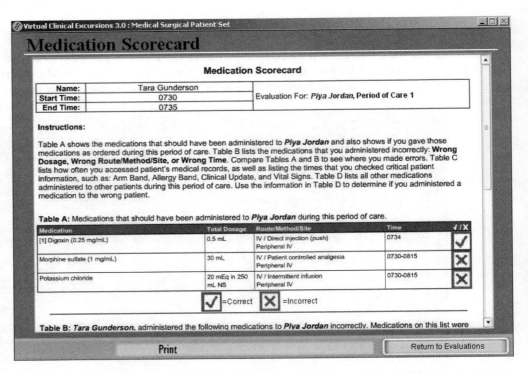

Not every medication listed on the MAR should be given. For example, a patient might have an allergy to a drug that was ordered, or a medication might have been improperly transcribed to the MAR. Predetermined medication "errors" embedded within the program challenge you to exercise critical thinking skills and professional judgment when deciding to administer a medication, just as you would in a real hospital. Use all your available resources, such as the patient's chart and the MAR, to make your decision.

Table C lists the resources that were available to assist you in medication administration, and it documents whether and when you accessed these resources. For example, did you check the patient armband or perform a check of vital signs? If so, when?

You can click **Print** to get a copy of this report if needed. Click **Return to Evaluations** when finished.

■ FLOOR MAP

To get a general sense of your location within the hospital, click on the **Map** icon found in the lower right corner of most of the screens in the *Virtual Clinical Excursions—Medical-Surgical* program. A floor map will appear, showing the layout of the floor you are currently on, as well as a directory of the patients and services on that floor. As you move your cursor over the directory list, the location of each room is highlighted (and vice versa). The floor map can be accessed from the Nurses' Station, Medication Room, and each patient's room.

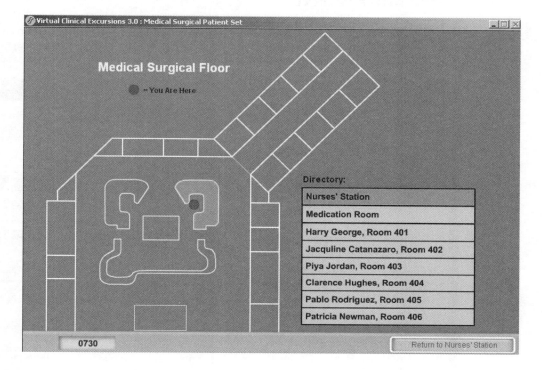

A DETAILED TOUR

If you wish to more thoroughly understand the capabilities of *Virtual Clinical Excursions—Medical-Surgical*, take a detailed tour by completing the following section. During this tour, we will work with a specific patient to introduce you to all the different components and learning opportunities available within the software.

■ WORKING WITH A PATIENT

Sign in and select the Medical-Surgical floor for Period of Care 1 (0730-0815). From the Patient List, select Piya Jordan in Room 403; however, do not go to the Nurses' Station yet.

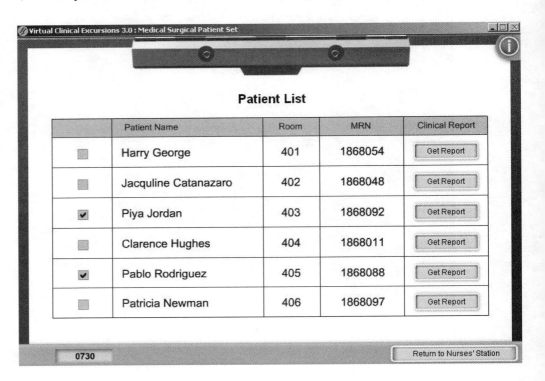

■ REPORT

In hospitals, when one shift ends and another begins, the outgoing nurse who attended a patient will give a verbal and sometimes a written summary of that patient's condition to the incoming nurse who will assume care for the patient. This summary is called a report and is an important source of data to provide an overview of a patient. Your first task is to get clinical report on Piya Jordan. To do this, click **Get Report** in the far right column in this patient's row. From this summary, identify the problems and areas of concern that you will need to address for this patient.

When you have finished reading the report and noting any areas of concern, click **Go to Nurses' Station**.

■ CHARTS

You can access Piya Jordan's chart from the Nurses' Station or from the patient's room (403). We will access it from the Nurses' Station: Click on the chart rack or on the **Chart** icon in the tool bar at the top of your screen. Next, click on the chart labeled **403** to open the medical record for Piya Jordan. Click on the **Emergency Department** tab to view a record of why this patient was admitted.

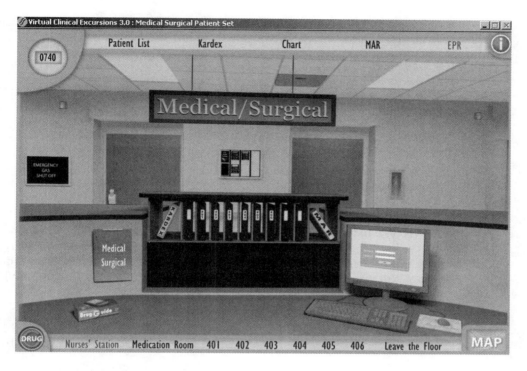

How many days has Piya Jordan been in the hospital?

What tests were done upon her arrival in the Emergency Department and why?

What was her reason for admission?

You should also click on **Surgical Reports** to learn what procedures were performed and when. Finally, review the **Nursing Admission** and **History and Physical** tabs to view information on the health history of this patient. When you are done reviewing the chart, click **Return to Nurses' Station**.

■ MEDICATIONS

Open the Medication Administration Record (MAR) by clicking on the **MAR** icon in the tool bar at the top of your screen. *Remember:* The MAR automatically opens to the first occupied room number on the floor (in this case, Room 401, Harry George). Since you need to access Piya Jordan's MAR, click on tab **403** (her room number). Always make sure you are giving the *Right Drug to the Right Patient!*

Examine the list of medications prescribed for Piya Jordan. Write down the medications that need to be given during this period of care (0730-0815). For each medication, note the dosage, route, and time in the chart below.

Time	Medication	Dosage	Route
0800	Digoxin	0.125 mg	IV

Click on **Return to Nurses' Station**. Next, click on **403** on the bottom tool bar and then verify that you are indeed in Piya Jordan's room. Select **Clinical Alerts** (the icon to the right of Initial Observations) to check for any emerging data that might affect your medication administration priorities. Go to the patient's chart (click on the **Chart** icon; then click on **403**). When the chart opens, select the **Physician's Orders** tab.

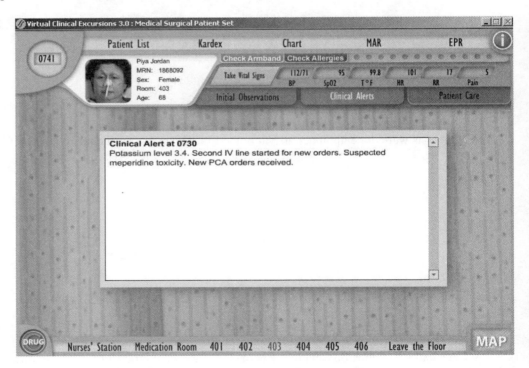

Review the orders. Have any new medications been ordered? Return to the MAR (click **Return to Room 403**; then click **MAR**). Verify that the new medications have been correctly transcribed to the MAR. Mistakes are sometimes made in the transcription process in the hospital setting, and it is sound practice to double-check any new order.

Are there any patient assessments you will need to perform before administering these medications? If so, return to Room 403 and click on **Review of Systems** to complete those before proceeding. (*Hint:* Check apical pulse.)

Now click on the **Medication Room** icon in the tool bar at the bottom of your screen to locate and prepare the medications for Piya Jordan.

In the Medication Room, you must access the medications for Piya Jordan from the specific dispensing system in which each medication is stored. Locate each medication that needs to be given in this time period and click on **Put Medication on Tray** as appropriate. (*Hint:* Look in Unit Dosage drawer first.) When you are finished, click on **Close Drawer** and then on **View Medication Room**. Now click on the medication tray on the counter on the left side of the medication room screen to begin preparing the medications you have selected. (*Note:* Instead of clicking on the tray, you can click **Preparation** at top of screen.)

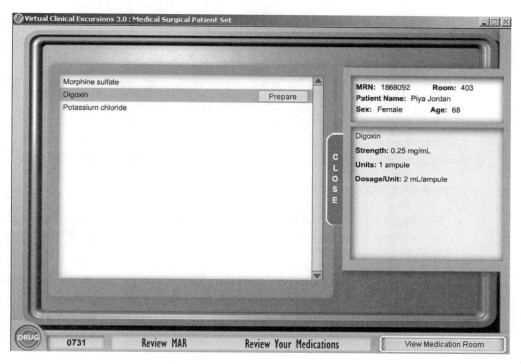

In the preparation area, you should see a list of the medications you put on the tray in the previous steps. Click on the first medication and then click **Prepare**. Follow the onscreen instructions of the Preparation Wizard, providing any data requested. As an example, let's follow the preparation process for digoxin, one of the medications due to be administered to Piya Jordan during this period of care. To begin, click to select **Digoxin**; then click **Prepare**. Now work through the Preparation Wizard sequence as detailed below:

> Amount of medication in the ampule: 2 mL
> Enter the amount of medication you will draw up into a syringe: **0.5** mL
> Click **Next**.
> Select the patient you wish to set aside the medication for:
> Click **Room 403, Piya Jordan**.
> Click **Finish**.
> Click **Return to Medication Room**.

Follow this same basic process for the other medications due to be administered to Piya Jordan during this period of care. (*Hint:* Look in **IV Storage** and **Automated System**.)

Preparation Wizard Exceptions

- Some medications in *Virtual Clinical Excursions—Medical-Surgical* are preprepared by the pharmacy (e.g., IV antibiotics) and taken to the patient room as a whole. This is common practice in most hospitals.
- Blood products are not administered by students through the *Virtual Clinical Excursions—Medical-Surgical* simulations since blood administration follows specific protocols not covered in this program.
- The *Virtual Clinical Excursions—Medical-Surgical* simulations do not allow for mixing more than one type of medication, such as regular and Lente insulins, in the same syringe. In the clinical setting, when multiple types of insulin are ordered for a patient, the regular insulin is drawn up first, followed by the longer-acting insulin. Insulin is always administered in a special unit-marked syringe.

Now return to Room 403 (click on **403** on bottom tool bar) to administer Piya Jordan's medications.

At any time during the medication administration process, you can perform a further review of systems, take vital signs, check information contained within the chart, or verify patient identity and allergies. Inside Piya Jordan's room, click **Take Vital Signs**. (*Note:* These findings change over time to reflect the temporal changes you would find in a patient similar to Piya Jordan.)

When you have gathered all the data you need, click on **Patient Care** and then select **Medication Administration**. After reviewing your medications, continue the administration process with the digoxin ordered for Piya Jordan. In the list of medications set aside for this patient, click to highlight **Digoxin**. Next, click on the down arrow to the right of **Select** and choose **Administer** from the drop-down menu. This will activate the Administration Wizard. Complete the Wizard sequence as follows:

- Route: **IV**
- Method: **Direct Injection**
- Site: **Peripheral IV**
- Click **Administer to Patient** arrow.
- Would you like to document this administration in the MAR? **Yes**
- Click **Finish** arrow.

Selections are recorded by a tracking system and evaluated on a Medication Scorecard stored under Preceptor's Evaluations. This scorecard can be viewed, printed, and given to your instructor. To access the Preceptor's Evaluations, click on **Leave the Floor**. When the Floor Menu appears, click on the icon next to **Look at Your Preceptor's Evaluation**. From the list of evaluations, click on **Medication Scorecard** inside the box with Piya Jordan's name.

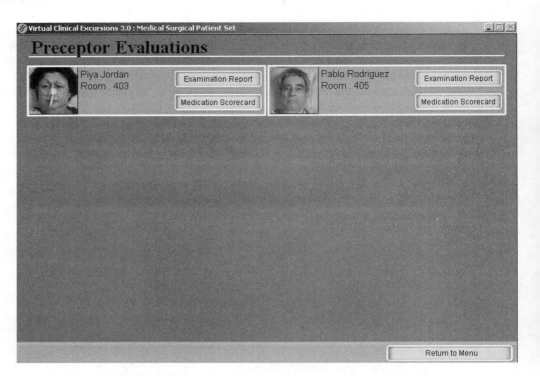

■ MEDICATION SCORECARD

- First, review Table A. Was digoxin given correctly? Did you give the other medications as ordered?
- Table B shows you which (if any) medications you gave incorrectly.
- Table C addresses the resources used for Piya Jordan. Did you access the patient's chart, MAR, EPR, or Kardex as needed to make safe medication administration decisions?
- Did you check the patient's armband to verify her identity? Did you check whether your patient had any known allergies to medications? Were vital signs taken?

Now that you understand the basic steps of medication preparation and administration, the following section will allow you to practice these skills further—with an increased emphasis on reducing medication errors by using the Medication Scorecard to evaluate your work.

■ REDUCING MEDICATION ERRORS: SELF-EVALUATION

Sign in to work at Pacific View Regional Hospital for Period of Care 1. (*Note:* If you are already working with another patient or during another period of care, click on **Leave the Floor** and then **Restart the Program**; then sign in.)

From the Patient List, select Clarence Hughes. Then click on **Go To Nurses' Station**. Complete the following steps to prepare and administer medications to Clarence Hughes.

- Click on **Medication Room**.
- Click on **MAR** to determine prn medications that have been ordered for Clarence Hughes to address his constipation and pain. (*Note:* You may click on **Review MAR** at any time to verify correct medication order. Remember to look at the patient name on the MAR to make sure you have the correct patient's record—you must click on the correct room number within the MAR.) Click on **Return to Medication Room** after reviewing the correct MAR.
- Click on **Unit Dosage** (or on the Unit Dosage cabinet); from the close-up view, click on drawer **404**.
- Select the medications you would like to administer. After each selection, click **Put Medication on Tray**. When you are finished selecting medications, click **Close Drawer**.
- Click on **View Medication Room**.
- Click on **Automated System** (or on the Automated System unit itself). Click **Login**.
- On the next screen, specify the correct patient and drawer location.
- Select the medication you would like to administer and click on **Put Medication on Tray**. Repeat this process if you wish to administer other medications from the Automated System.
- When you are finished, click **Close Drawer**. At the bottom right corner of the next screen, click on **View Medication Room**.
- From the Medication Room, click on **Preparation** (or on the preparation tray).
- From the list of medications on your tray, choose the correct medication to administer.
- Click **Next**, specify the correct patient to administer this medication to, and click **Finish**.
- Repeat the previous two steps until all medications that you want to administer are prepared.
- You can click on **Review Your Medications** and then on **Return to Medication Room** when ready. Once you are back in the Medication Room, go directly to Clarence Hughes' room by clicking on **404** at bottom of screen.
- Inside the patient's room, administer the medication, utilizing the five rights of medication administration. After you have collected the appropriate assessment data and are ready for administration, click **Patient Care** and then **Medication Administration**. Verify that the correct patient and medication(s) appear in the left-hand window. Then click the down arrow next to Select. From the drop-down menu, select **Administer** and complete the Administration Wizard by providing any information requested. When the Wizard stops asking for information, click **Administer to Patient**. Specify **Yes** when asked whether this administration should be recorded in the MAR. Finally, click **Finish**.

Now let's see how you did during your earlier medication administration!

- Click on **Leave the Floor** at the bottom of your screen. From the Floor Menu, select **Look at Your Preceptor's Evaluation**. Then click on **Medication Scorecard**.

These resources will help you find out more about each patient's medications and possible sources of medication errors.

1. Start by examining Table A. These are the medications you should have given to Clarence Hughes during this period of care. If each of the medications in Table A has a √ by it, then you made no errors. Congratulations!

If there are some medications that have an X by them, then you made one or more medication errors.

Compare Tables A and B to determine which of the following types of errors you made: Wrong Dose, Wrong Route/Method/Site, or Wrong Time. Follow these steps:
   a. Find medications in Table A that were given incorrectly.
   b. Now see if those same medications are in Table B, which shows what you actually administered to Clarence Hughes.
   c. Comparing Tables A and B, match the Strength, Dose, Route/Method/Site, and Time for each medication you administered incorrectly.
   d. Then, using the form below, list the medications given incorrectly and mark the errors you made for each medication.

Medication	Strength	Dosage	Route	Method	Site	Time
	❑	❑	❑	❑	❑	❑
	❑	❑	❑	❑	❑	❑
	❑	❑	❑	❑	❑	❑
	❑	❑	❑	❑	❑	❑

2. To help you reduce future medication errors, consider the following list of possible reasons for errors.

   • Did not check drug against MAR for correct patient, correct date, correct time, correct drug, and correct dose.
   • Did not check drug dose against MAR three times.
   • Did not open the unit dose package in the patient's room.
   • Did not correctly identify the patient using two identifiers.
   • Did not administer the drug on time.
   • Did not verify patient allergies.
   • Did not check the patient's current condition or vital sign parameters.
   • Did not consider why the patient would be receiving this drug.
   • Did not question why the drug was in the patient's drawer.
   • Did not check the physician's order and/or check with the pharmacist when there was a question about the drug or dose.
   • Did not verify that no adverse effects had occurred from a previous dose.

Based on these possibilities, determine how you made each error and record the reason into the form below:

Medication	Reason for Error

3. Look again at Table B. Are there medications listed that are not in Table A? If so, you gave a medication to Clarence Hughes that he should not have received. Complete the following exercises to help you understand how such an error might have been made.

   a. Perhaps you gave a medication that was on Clarence Hughes' MAR for this period of care, without recognizing that a change had occurred in the patient's condition that should have caused you to reconsider. Review patient records as necessary and complete the following form:

Medication	Possible Reasons Not to Give This Medication

   b. Another possibility is that you gave Clarence Hughes a medication that should have been given at a different time. Check his MAR and complete the form below to determine whether you made a Wrong Time error:

Medication	Given to Clarence Hughes at What Time	Should Have Been Given at What Time

c. Maybe you gave another patient's medication to Clarence Hughes. In this case, you made a Wrong Patient error. Check the MARs of other patients and use the form below to determine whether you made this type of error:

Medication	Given to Clarence Hughes	Should Have Been Given to

4. The Medication Scorecard provides some other interesting sources of information. For example, if there is a medication selected for Clarence Hughes but it was not given to him, there will be an X by that medication in Table A, but it will not appear in Table B. In that case, you might have given this medication to some other patient, which is another type of Wrong Patient error. To investigate further, look at Table D, which lists the medications you gave to other patients. See whether you can find any medications for Clarence Hughes that were given to another patient by mistake. Before making any decisions, be sure to cross-check the other patients' MAR because they may have had the same medication ordered. Use the following form to record your findings:

Medication	Should Have Been Given to Clarence Hughes	Given by Mistake to

5. Now take some time to review the exercises you just completed. Use the form below to create an overall analysis of what you have learned. Once again, record each of the medication errors you made, including the type of each error. Then, for each error you made, indicate specifically what you would do differently to prevent this type of error from occurring again.

Medication	Type of Error	Error Prevention Tactic

Submit this form to your instructor if required as a graded assignment, or simply use these exercises to improve your understanding of medication errors and how to reduce them.

Name: _____   Date: _____

■ **VITAL SIGNS**

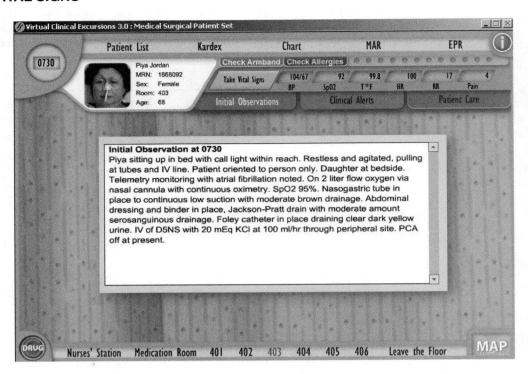

Vital signs, often considered the traditional signs of life, include body temperature, heart rate, respiratory rate, blood pressure, oxygen saturation of the blood, and the patient's experience of pain.

Inside Piya Jordan's room, click **Take Vital Signs**. (*Remember:* You can take vital signs at any time. The data change over time to reflect the temporal changes you would find in a patient similar to Piya Jordan.) Collect vital signs for this patient and record them in the following table. Note the time at which you collected each of these data.

Vital Signs	Findings/Time
Blood pressure	
O$_2$ saturation	
Heart rate	
Respiratory rate	
Temperature	
Pain rating	

After you are done, click on the **EPR** icon located in the tool bar at the top of the screen.

Complete the EPR Login screen as directed in *A Quick Tour* (see page 15 of this workbook). Click on the down arrow next to Patient and choose Piya Jordan's room number **403**. Select **Vital Signs** as the category. Next, record the vital signs data you just collected in the last column. (*Note:* If you need help with this process, see page 16.) Now compare these findings with the data you collected earlier for this patient's vital signs. Use these earlier findings to establish a baseline for each of the vital signs.

      a.   Are any of the data you collected significantly different from the baseline for a particular vital sign?

          Circle One: Yes   No

      b.   If "Yes," which data are different?

■ PHYSICAL ASSESSMENT

After you have finished examining the EPR for vital signs, click **Exit EPR** to return to Room 403. Click **Patient Care** and then **Physical Assessment**. Think about what information you received in report, as well as what you may have learned about this patient from the chart. What area(s) of examination should you pay most attention to at this time? Is there any equipment you should be monitoring? Conduct a physical assessment of the body areas and systems that you consider priorities for Piya Jordan. For example, select **Head & Neck**; then click on and assess **Mental Status** and **Equipment**. Complete any other assessment(s) you think are necessary at this time. In the following table, record the data you collected during this examination.

Area of Examination	Findings
Head & Neck Mental Status	
Head & Neck Equipment	

After you have finished collecting these data, return to the EPR. Compare the data that were already in the record with those you just collected.

    a.   Are any of the data you collected significantly different from the baselines for this patient?

        Circle One: Yes   No

    b.   If "Yes," which data are different?

■ NURSE-CLIENT INTERACTIONS

Click on **Patient Care** from inside Piya Jordan's room (403). Now click on **Nurse-Client Interactions** to access a short video titled **Pain—Adverse Drug Event**, which is available for viewing at 0735 (based on the virtual clock in the upper left corner of your screen). To begin the video, click on the arrow next to its title. You will observe a nurse communicating with Piya Jordan and her daughter. There are many variations of nursing practice, some exemplifying "best" practice and some not. Note whether the nurse in this interaction displays professional behavior and compassionate care. Are her words congruent with what is going on with the patient? Does this interaction "feel right" to you? If not, how would you handle this situation differently? Explain.

Note: If the video you wish to view is not listed, this means you have not yet reached the correct virtual time to view that video. Check the virtual clock; you may return to access the video once its designated time has occurred—as long as you do so within the corresponding period of care.

At least one Nurse-Client Interactions video is available during each period of care. Viewing these videos can help you learn more about what is occurring with a patient at a certain time and also prompt you to discriminate between nurse communications that are ideal and those that need improvement. Compassionate care and the ability to communicate clearly are essential components of delivering quality nursing care, and it is during your clinical time that you will begin to refine these skills.

■ COLLECTING AND EVALUATING DATA

Each of the activities you perform in the Patient Care environment generates a great deal of assessment data. Remember that after you collect data, you can record your findings in the EPR. You can also review the EPR, patient's chart, videos, and MAR at any time. You will get plenty of practice collecting and then evaluating data in context of the patient's course.

Now, here's an important question for you:

> Did the previous sequence of exercises provide the most efficient way to assess Piya Jordan?

For example, you went to the patient's room to get vital signs, then back to the EPR to enter data and compare your findings with extant data. Next, you went back to the patient's room to do a physical examination, then again back to the EPR to enter and review data. If this back-and-forth process of data collection and recording seemed inefficient, remember the following:

- Plan all of your nursing activities to maximize efficiency while at the same time optimizing quality of patient care. (Think about what data you might need to perform certain tasks. For example, do you need to check a heart rate before administering a cardiac medication or check an IV site before starting an infusion?)

- You collect a tremendous amount of data when you work with a patient. Very few people can accurately remember all these data for more than a few minutes. Develop efficient assessment skills, and record data as soon as possible after collecting them.

- Assessment data are only the starting point for the nursing process.

Make a clear distinction between these first exercises and how you actually provide nursing care. These initial exercises were designed to involve you actively in the use of different software components. This workbook focuses on sensible practices for implementing the nursing process in ways that ensure the highest quality care of patients.

Most important, remember that a human being changes through time, and that these changes include both the physical and psychosocial facets of a person as a living organism. Think about this for a moment. Some patients may change physically in a very short time (a patient with emerging myocardial infarction) or more slowly (a patient with a chronic illness). Patients' overall physical and psychosocial conditions may improve or deteriorate. They may have effective coping skills and familial support, or they may feel alone and full of despair. In fact, each individual is a complex mix of physical and psychosocial elements, and at least some of these elements usually change through time.

Thus it is crucial *not* to think of the nursing process as a simple one-time, five-step procedure:

- Assessment
- Nursing Diagnosis
- Planning
- Implementation
- Evaluation

Rather, the nursing process should be utilized as a creative and systematic approach to delivering nursing care. Furthermore, because all living organisms are constantly changing, we must apply the nursing process over and over. Each time we follow the nursing process for an individual patient, we refine our understanding of that patient's physical and psychosocial conditions based on collection and analysis of many different types of data. *Virtual Clinical Excursions—Medical-Surgical* will help you develop both the creativity and the systematic approach needed to become a nurse who is equipped to deliver the highest quality care to all patients.

The following icons are used throughout the workbook to help you quickly identify particular activities and assignments:

 Indicates a reading assignment—tells you which textbook chapter(s) you should read before starting each lesson

 Indicates a writing activity

 Marks the beginning of an interactive CD-ROM activity—signals you to open or return to your *Virtual Clinical Excursions—Medical-Surgical* CD-ROM

 Indicates additional CD-ROM instructions

 Indicates questions and activities that require you to consult your textbook

 Indicates the approximate time required to complete an exercise

LESSON **1**

Health Assessment

 Reading Assignment: Health Assessment (Chapter 4)

Patients: Piya Jordan, Room 403
Clarence Hughes, Room 404
Pablo Rodiguez, Room 405

Goal: Accurately obtain a complete health assessment.

Objectives:

1. Describe appropriate guidelines for the health history interview.
2. Obtain a complete health history of an assigned patient.
3. Prioritize data collection from a patient in an acute situation.
4. Describe the four primary techniques utilized in physical examination.
5. Perform and document a thorough physical examination on an assigned patient.

In this lesson you will discuss and obtain a complete health assessment on assigned patients. Begin this activity by reviewing the general concepts presented in your textbook. Answer the following questions to solidify your understanding of culture.

Exercise 1

Clinical Preparation: Writing Activity

20 minutes

1. What environmental factors are most conducive for a health history interview?

2. Describe appropriate guidelines related to the patient when conducting a health history interview.

3. Describe appropriate guidelines related to the interviewer when conducting a health history interview.

4. Identify the five major components of the health history.

5. Document and describe the four primary techniques utilized in a physical assessment by completing the table below.

Technique	Description
a.	
b.	
c.	
d.	

Exercise 2

 CD-ROM Activity

 30 minutes

- Sign in to work at Pacific View Regional Hospital for Period of Care 1. (*Note:* If you are already in the virtual hospital from a previous exercise, click on **Leave the Floor** and then **Restart the Program** to get to the sign-in window.)
- From the Patient List, select Piya Jordan (Room 403) and Pablo Rodriguez (Room 405).
- Click on **Go to Nurses' Station**.
- Click on **403** to go to Piya Jordan's room.

1. As a student nurse, you are entering the patient's room to obtain a health history for your assigned clinical preparation documentation. What do you learn about Piya Jordan's state of mind from the initial observation?

2. Can you obtain an accurate history from Piya Jordan at this time? Why or why not?

3. You know that your instructor will still expect you to know Piya Jordan's current history. Other than reading the physician's H&P, how could you obtain this information?

→ • Click on **Nurses' Station**.
 • Click on **Chart** and then on **405** to obtain Pablo Rodriguez's record.
 • Click on **Nursing Admission**.

4. Health assessment begins with the health history. You will now document a health history on Pablo Rodriguez, using the long format discussed in your textbook. This format differs from that used in the Pacific View Regional Hospital chart on your CD-ROM. Read the Nursing Admission form to obtain and record the information requested below and on the next four pages. If the information is not available, write N/A.

Biographic Data

Current Health
     Chief complaint

     Symptom analysis

Past Health History

Family Health History

Psychosocial History
     Psychosocial risk factors
          Social history

          Personal and family history

          Level of stress

Usual coping pattern

Changes in neurophysiologic function

Level of understanding about health problems

Mental status

Personality style

Major psychosocial reactions

Psychologic Assessment
  General appearance

Motor activity

Behavior

Mental status

Level of consciousness

Orientation to person, place, time, and circumstances

Mood and affect

Speech and communication (language)

Thought process and content

Attention span

Memory: immediate, recent, and remote

General fund of knowledge

Calculations

Abstract reasoning and thinking

Perceptual distortion

Judgment

Insight

Other Psychologic Factors
   Motivation

Personal strengths

Values and beliefs

Spirituality

Sociologic Assessment
    Psychosocial development

    Social network

    Socioeconomic status

    Lifestyle

    Sexuality

Cultural Asssessment

Review of Systems
    Neurologic

    Musculoskeletal

    Cardiovascular

    Respiratory

    Integumentary

Gastrointestinal

Genitourinary

Health Risk Appraisal

5. Compare your health history format with the one used in the chart on your CD-ROM. Which format do you believe directs the nurse to obtain the most complete health history? Explain.

Exercise 3

 CD-ROM Activity

 40 minutes

- Sign in to work at Pacific View Regional Hospital for Period of Care 2. (*Note:* If you are already in the virtual hospital from a previous exercise, click on **Leave the Floor** and then **Restart the Program** to get to the sign-in window.)
- From the Patient List, select Clarence Hughes (Room 404) and Pablo Rodriguez (Room 405).
- Click on **Go to Nurses' Station**.
- Click on **404** to enter Clarence Hughes' room.

1. As a student nurse, you are entering Clarence Hughes' room to obtain a health history for your assigned clinical preparation documentation. What do you learn about Clarence Hughes from the initial observation?

2. Would it be appropriate to obtain a complete history at this time? If not, how would you adapt your data collection at this point? (*Hint:* See page 68 in your textbook.)

- Click on **405** to enter Pablo Rodriguez's room.
- Click on **Patient Care**.

3. Health assessment continues with the physical examination. You will now perform a head-to-toe assessment on Pablo Rodriguez. For each of the main body areas listed in the table below and on the next three pages, click on the corresponding yellow button on your screen. Then select each of the assessment subcategories and record your findings in the middle column of the table. (*Note:* You will complete the table in questions 4 and 5.)

Area Assessed	Assessment Findings	Technique(s) Used
Head & Neck Sensory		
Lymphatic		
Musculoskeletal		
Gastrointestinal		
Neurologic		
Thyroid		

Area Assessed	Assessment Findings	Technique(s) Used
Integumentary		
Mental Status		
Chest Integumentary		
Cardiovascular		
Breasts		
Respiratory		
Musculoskeletal		
Back & Spine Integumentary		
Musculoskeletal		
Respiratory		
Upper Extremities Integumentary		

Area Assessed	Assessment Findings	Technique(s) Used
Musculoskeletal		
Vascular		
Neurologic		
Abdomen		
Integumentary		
Musculoskeletal		
Gastrointestinal		
Reproductive		
Pelvic		
Integumentary		
Gastrointestinal		
Urologic		
Reproductive		

Area Assessed	Assessment Findings	Technique(s) Used
Lower Extremities Integumentary		
Musculoskeletal		
Vascular		
Neurologic		

4. Identify the technique(s) of examination that would be used to obtain each of the findings you recorded in the table in question 3. Document these techniques in the last column of the table.

5. Review the physical examination data collected in question 3. Place an asterisk (*) next to any abnormal assessment data.

6. Based on the abnormal data identified in question 5, summarize Pablo Rodriguez's health problems.

7. Identify two priority nursing diagnosis for Pablo Rodriguez.

LESSON 2

Fluid Imbalance

Reading Assignment: Clients with Fluid Imbalances (Chapter 13)

Patients: Piya Jordan, Room 403
Patricia Newman, Room 406

Goal: Utilize the nursing process to competently care for patients with fluid imbalances.

Objectives:

1. Identify normal physiologic influences on fluid and electrolyte balance.
2. Compare and contrast the pathophysiology related to dehydration and overhydration.
3. Utilize laboratory data and clinical manifestations to assess fluid balance and imbalance.
4. Describe collaborative management strategies used to maintain and/or restore fluid balance.
5. Critically analyze differences in fluid balance assessment findings between different patients.
6. Develop an appropriate plan of care for patients displaying fluid imbalances.

In this lesson you will assess, plan, and implement care for two patients with similar but differing fluid imbalances. Piya Jordan is a 68-year-old female admitted with nausea and vomiting for several days following weeks of poor appetite and increasing weakness. Patricia Newman is a 61-year-old female admitted with dyspnea at rest, cough, and fever. You will begin this activity by reviewing the general concepts of fluid homeostasis as presented in your textbook. Answer the following questions to cement your understanding of the normal physiologic concepts related to fluid balance.

Exercise 1

 Clinical Preparation: Writing Activity

 30 minutes

1. Describe the two fluid compartments in the body and describe their composition.

2. Compare and contrast the causes and clinical manifestations of various types of fluid imbalances by completing the table below and on the next page.

Fluid Imbalance	Causes	Clinical Manifestations
Extracellular fluid volume deficit (ECFVD) (Dehydration)		
Intracellular fluid volume deficit (Cellular dehydration)		
Extracellular fluid volume excess (ECFVE) (Hypervolemia)		

Fluid Imbalance	Causes	Clinical Manifestations
Intracellular fluid volume excess (ICFVE) (Water intoxication)		
Extracellular fluid volume shift: third-spacing		

Exercise 2

  CD-ROM Activity

 40 minutes

- Sign in to work at Pacific View Regional Hospital for Period of Care 1. (*Note:* If you are already in the virtual hospital from a previous exercise, click on **Leave the Floor** and then **Restart the Program** to get to the sign-in window.)
- From the Patient List, select Piya Jordan (Room 403).
- Click on **Go to Nurses' Station**.
- Click on **Chart** and then on **403** for Piya Jordan's chart.
- Click on **Emergency Department** and review this record.

  1. Record findings below that support the diagnosis of dehydration.

→ • Click on **Nursing Admission**.

  2. Are there any additional findings noted on this document that support the diagnosis of dehydration? If so, list them below.

➡ • Click on **Laboratory Reports**.

3. Below, record pertinent results noted on Piya Jordan's admission (Monday at 2200) and describe the significance of each result in relation to the diagnosis of dehydration.

 4. Calculate Piya Jordan's plasma osmolality, using the more accurate formula described in Box 13-1 of the textbook.

5. Based on the above findings, what type of dehydration do you think Piya Jordan is suffering from? (*Hint:* See pages 207-208 of the textbook.) Explain.

➡ • Click on **History and Physical**.

6. What were the contributing factors leading to this dehydration?

➡ • Click on **Physician's Orders**.

7. Identify orders that are appropriate management strategies for the treatment of dehydration.

Exercise 3

 CD-ROM Activity

 45 minutes

Now you will answer similar questions related to fluid balance for another patient and compare the findings.

- Sign in to work at Pacific View Regional Hospital for Period of Care 1. (*Note:* If you are already in the virtual hospital from a previous exercise, click on **Leave the Floor** and then **Restart the Program** to get to the sign-in window.)
- From the Patient List, select Patricia Newman (Room 406).
- Click on **Go to Nurse's Station**.
- Click on **Chart** and then on **406** for Patricia Newman's chart.
- Click on **Emergency Department** and review this record.

  1. Identify assessment findings related to fluid balance and record below. How do these findings differ from those for Piya Jordan? Are there any similarities?

 • Click on **Nursing Admission**.

  2. Are there any additional findings noted on this document related to fluid balance and/or imbalance? If so, list them below. How do they compare with findings for Piya Jordan?

 • Click on **Laboratory Results**.

  3. Record pertinent results below and describe the significance of each result in relation to fluid balance, Describe any differences between these findings and those for Piya Jordan.

4. Calculate Patricia Newman's plasma osmolality (again using the more accurate formula described in Box 13-1 of the textbook). Is the result decreased, normal, or elevated?

5. Based on the above findings, does Patricia Newman have a fluid imbalance? Is so, what type?

→ • Click on **History and Physical**.

6. What are the contributing factors for this patient's potential or actual fluid imbalance?

7. What coexisting illness might have an impact on the selection and rate of IV fluid therapy?

8. Develop an appropriate plan of care for patients with either fluid volume deficit or fluid volume excess by completing the table below.

Collaborative Plan of Care	Fluid Volume Deficit	Fluid Volume Excess
Patient outcomes		
Assessment parameters		
Interventions		

LESSON 3

Electrolyte Imbalance, Part 1

📖 **Reading Assignment:** Clients with Electrolyte Imbalances (Chapter 14)

Patients: Piya Jordan, Room 403
Patricia Newman, Room 406

Goal: Utilize the nursing process to competently care for patients with electrolyte imbalances.

Objectives:

1. Describe the effect of potassium imbalances on the action potential.
2. Identify specific etiologic factors related to hypokalemia for assigned patients.
3. Research potential drug interactions related to hypokalemia for assigned patients.
4. Assess patients for clinical manifestations related to hypo- and hyperkalemia.
5. Utilize the nursing process to correctly administer IV potassium chloride per physician's orders.

In this lesson you will assess, plan, and implement care for two patients with hypokalemia. Piya Jordan is a 68-year-old female admitted with nausea and vomiting for several days following weeks of poor appetite and increasing weakness. Patricia Newman is a 61-year-old female admitted with pneumonia and a history of emphysema for 12 years. You will begin this activity by reviewing the general functions of electrolytes within the body as presented in your textbook. Answer the following questions to cement your understanding of the normal physiologic concepts related to potassium balance.

Exercise 1

✏️ **Clinical Preparation: Writing Activity**

 30 minutes

1. Cells use electrolytes for what two main purposes?

2. Describe the effect of potassium imbalance on the action potential.

3. Identify causes and/or risk factors for hypokalemia.

4. Describe the clinical manifestations associated with hypokalemia.

5. Identify causes and/or risk factors for hyperkalemia.

6. Describe the clinical manifestations associated with hyperkalemia.

Exercise 2

 CD-ROM Activity

 45 minutes

- Sign in to work at Pacific View Regional Hospital for Period of Care 1. (*Note:* If you are already in the virtual hospital from a previous exercise, click on **Leave the Floor** and then **Restart the Program** to get to the sign-in window.)
- From the Patient List, select Piya Jordan (Room 403).
- Click on **Go to Nurses' Station**.
- Click on **Chart** and then on **403**.
- Click on the **Laboratory Reports** tab.

1. What was Piya Jordan's initial potassium level on Monday at 2200?

 • Click on **Emergency Department** and review this record.

2. What would be the most likely cause for hypokalemia in this patient?

3. What did the physician order to treat this electrolyte imbalance? Is this appropriate? Is the dilution and rate safe to administer to Piya Jordan? Explain your answer. (*Hint:* If you need help, return to the Nurses' Station and click on the **Drug Guide** on the counter or click on the **Drug** icon in the bottom left corner of your screen.)

4. What precautions should be taken when administering the above IV solution of potassium?

→ • Click again on **Laboratory Reports**.

5. What was Piya Jordan's potassium level for Tuesday at 0630? Was the physician's order for potassium effective? Is there any cause for concern?

→ • Click on **Return to Nurses' Station**.
   • Go to Room **403**.
   • Click on **Patient Care**.

6. Complete a physical assessment on Piya Jordan, specifically looking for clinical manifestations of hypokalemia. Document your findings in the chart below and place an asterisk (*) next to those that correlate with hypokalemia.

Areas Assessed	Findings on Physical Examination
Cardiovascular	
Respiratory	
Neuromuscular	
Gastrointestinal	
Renal	

7. What is the potassium level that was drawn on Wednesday at 0630?

8. Explain the etiology for this recurrence of hypokalemia.

• Go to the **Chart**.
- Click on **Physician's Orders**.

9. What did the physician order for Piya Jordan in response to today's potassium level?

Prepare to administer this ordered dose of potassium chloride to Piya Jordan by completing the following steps.

Medication Preparation

 • Click on **Return to Room 403**.
- Click **Medication Room** on the bottom of your screen.
- Click on **IV Storage** near the top of your screen (*Note:* You can also click on any of the three bins just above the refrigerator.) Either of these methods will bring up a close-up view of the IV storage bins.
- Click on the bin labeled **Small Volume** and review the list of available medications. (*Note:* You may click on **Review MAR** at any time to verify correct medication order. Remember to look at the patient name on the MAR to make sure you have the correct patient's record— you must click on the correct room number within the MAR. Click on **Return to Medication Room** after reviewing the correct MAR.)
- From the list of medications in the bin, select **potassium chloride**. Then click **Put Medication on Tray** and **Close Bin**.
- Click **View Medication Room**.
- Click on **Preparation** at the top of the screen or on the preparation tray on the counter. Select the correct medication to administer; then click **Prepare**.
- Wait for instructions or questions from the Preparation Wizard. Then click **Next**.
- Choose the correct patient to administer this medication to. Click **Finish**.
- You can click **Review Your Medications** and then **Return to Medication Room** when ready. From the Medication Room, go directly to Piya Jordan's room by clicking on **403** at bottom of screen.

Prior to administering intravenous medications, the patient's IV site must first be assessed.

 • Click on **Patient Care**.
- Click on **Upper Extremities**.
- Select **Integumentary** from the system subcategories.

10. Document the IV site assessment findings below. Is it appropriate to administer the IV potassium at this time?

Medication Administration

- After you have collected the appropriate assessment data and are ready for administration, click on **Medication Administration**. (*Note:* If you are not still in the Patient Care screen, you will need to first click **Patient Care** and then choose **Medication Administration**.)
- To the right of the medication name, next to Select, click the down arrow and choose **Administer** from the drop-down menu.
- Complete the Administration Wizard and click **Administer to Patient** when done.
- Check **Yes** when asked whether this drug administration should be documented on the MAR. Then click **Finish**.
- Now click on **MAR** at the top of your screen.

11. Look at Piya Jordan's MAR. What are her scheduled AM medications? What medication would you question giving? Why?

Now let's see how you did!

- Click on **Leave the Floor** at the bottom of your screen. From the Floor Menu, select **Look at Your Preceptor's Evaluation**. Then click on **Medication Scorecard**.

12. Disregard the report for the routine scheduled medications, but note below whether or not you correctly administered the potassium chloride. If not, why do you think you were incorrect in administering this drug? According to Table C in this scorecard, what are the appropriate resources that should be used and important assessments that should be completed prior to administering this medication? Did you use these resources and perform these assessments correctly?

Exercise 3

 CD-ROM Activity

 30 minutes

- Sign in to work at Pacific View Regional Hospital for Period of Care 1. (*Note:* If you are already in the virtual hospital from a previous exercise, click on **Leave the Floor** and then **Restart the Program** to get to the sign-in window.)
- From the Patient List, select Patricia Newman (Room 406).
- Click on **Go to Nurses' Station**.
- Click on **Charts** and then on **406**.
- Click on **Laboratory Reports**.

  1. What was Patricia Newman's initial potassium level this morning?

- Click on **History and Physical**.

  2. What would be the most likely cause for hypokalemia in this patient?

- Click on **Physician's Orders**.

  3. What did the physician order to treat this electrolyte imbalance?

- Click on **MAR**.

  4. What is missing from this order?

  5. Where could you verify this missing information?

6. What is the difference between the treatment of hypokalemia for Piya Jordan and that for Patricia Newman? Explain the difference.

 • Click on **Chart**.
   • Click on **Physician's Orders**.

7. Look again at the physician's orders. Is there an order for any follow-up lab work?

8. What is the nurse's responsibility in regard to follow-up lab work? How would you handle this situation?

 • Click on **Return to Nurses' Station**.
   • Click on **406** to go to Patricia Newman's room.
   • Click on **Patient Care**.
   • Click on **Nurse-Client Interactions**.
   • Select and view the video titled **0740: Evaluation—Response to Care**. (*Note:* If this video is not available, check the virtual clock to see whether enough time has elapsed. The video cannot be viewed before its specified time.)

9. Although Patricia Newman is happy that her chest does not hurt like it did, what does she verbalize as a concern?

10. What is the nurse's response to the patient's expressed concern?

11. When evaluating the care of Patricia Newman, for what potential complications of IV potassium therapy would you monitor? (*Hint:* For help, return to the Nurses' Station and click on the **Drug Guide** on the counter or click on the **Drug** icon in the bottom left corner of your screen.)

4

Electrolyte Imbalance, Part 2

/👓 **Reading Assignment:** Clients with Electrolyte Imbalances (Chapter 14)

Patient: Pablo Rodriguez, Room 405

Goal: Utilize the nursing process to competently care for patients with electrolyte imbalances.

Objectives:

1. Describe the pathophysiologic basis of electrolyte imbalances noted on a specific patient.
2. Identify specific etiologic factor(s) related to hypercalcemia, hyponatremia, and hypophosphatemia in the assigned patient.
3. Assess the assigned patient for clinical manifestations related to sodium, calcium, and phosphorus imbalances.
4. Describe nursing interventions appropriate when caring for a patient with hypercalcemia, hyponatremia, and hypophosphatemia.
5. Evaluate the effectiveness of medication prescribed to treat electrolyte imbalances.

In this lesson you will assess, plan, and implement care for a patient with several electrolyte imbalances. Pablo Rodriguez is a 71-year-old male who is admitted with nausea and vomiting for several days. He has a 1-year history of lung carcinoma. You will begin this activity by reviewing the general functions of specific electrolytes within the body as presented in your textbook. Answer the following questions to cement your understanding of the physiologic concepts related to phosphorous, sodium, and calcium imbalance.

73

Exercise 1

Clinical Preparation: Writing Activity

15 minutes

1. Prior to caring for a patient with multiple electrolyte imbalances, it is imperative that you first review and reinforce general concepts related to specific electrolytes. Using the textbook, complete the table below by providing information related to specific calcium, phosphorous, and sodium imbalances. Refer to this table as you proceed through the CD-ROM activity to relate textbook knowledge to actual patient care.

Electrolyte Imbalance	Lab Value	Etiology and Risk Factors	Pathophysiology
Hypercalcemia	>5.5 mEq/L or 11.0 mg/dL		
Hypophosphatemia	<1.2 mEq/L or 2.8 mg/dL		
Hyponatremia	<135 mEq/L		

Exercise 2

 CD-ROM Activity

 45 minutes

- Sign in to work at Pacific View Regional Hospital for Period of Care 1. (*Note:* If you are already in the virtual hospital from a previous exercise, click on **Leave the Floor** and then **Restart the Program** to get to the sign-in window.)
- From the Patient List, select Pablo Rodriguez (Room 405).
- Click on **Go to Nurses' Station**.
- Click on **Chart** at top of the screen or on the rack of charts in the center of the screen.
- Click on **405** to view Pablo Rodriguez's chart.
- Click on **Laboratory Reports**.

1. Record Pablo Rodriguez's serum chemistry results in the table below. Identify abnormal values by marking as H (for high) or L (for low). (*Hint:* Lab value results for calcium, phosphorous, and magnesium are measured in mg/dL.)

Laboratory Test	Laboratory Result Tuesday 2000	Laboratory Result Wednesday 0730
Sodium		
Potassium		
Calcium		
Phosphorous		
Magnesium		

 • Click on **Emergency Department**.

2. What would be the most likely cause for the hyponatremia noted on admission in this patient?

3. What did the physician order to treat this electrolyte imbalance?

4. What was Pablo Rodriguez's sodium level for Wednesday at 0730? Was the physician's ordered treatment effective? Are there any changes in physician orders you might anticipate or suggest?

5. Hyponatremia can be associated with both hypovolemia (actual sodium loss) and hypervolumia (dilutional). Initially, in the Emergency Department, what do you think Pablo Rodriguez's volume status was? Explain.

- Click on **Return to Nurses' Station**.
- Click on **EPR** and then on **Login**.
- Select **405** for the patient's room and **Intake and Output** as the category.

6. Record Pablo Rodriguez's I&O shift totals below.

Shift Totals	Tuesday 0705	Tuesday 1505	Tuesday 2305	Wednesday 0705
Intake				
Output				

7. On reviewing the above I&O totals obtained after the patient received IV replacement therapy, what factor(s) may be contributing to the persistant hyponatremia? Explain your answer.

8. What other lab tests might be useful to more accurately determine the patient's hydration status? (*Hint:* See page 215 of the textbook.)

- Click on **Return to Nurses' Station**.
- Click on **405** to go to the patient's room.
- Inside the room, click on **Patient Care**.

 9. Complete a physical assessment on Pablo Rodriguez, specifically looking for clinical manifestations of hyponatremia. (*Hint:* Refer to page 226 in your textbook.) Document your findings in the table below and place an asterisk (*) by those that correlate with hyponatremia.

Areas Assessed	Findings on Physical Examination
Cardiovascular	
Respiratory	
Neuromuscular	
Gastrointestinal	

- Click on **Chart**.
- Click on **Nursing Admission**.

10. Review the findings that you marked with an asterisk in question 9. What other factors noted on the Nursing Admission form could be causing or contributing to these manifestations?

11. Based on your answer to the last two questions, what conclusion can you make regarding these clinical manifestations and Pablo Rodriguez's sodium levels?

 12. What other clinical manifestations of hyponatremia might you expect to find in other patients with this electrolyte imbalance? (*Hint:* See page 226 in the textbook.)

13. If Pablo Rodriguez had a sodium level of 110 mEq/L (severe hyponatremia), how would the treatment vary?

Exercise 3

 CD-ROM Activity

60 minutes

- Sign in to work at Pacific View Regional Hospital for Period of Care 3. (*Note:* If you are already in the virtual hospital from a previous exercise, click on **Leave the Floor** and then **Restart the Program** to get to the sign-in window.)
- From the Patient List, select Pablo Rodriguez (Room 405).
- Click on **Go to Nurses' Station**.
- Click on **Chart** at the top of the screen.

- Click on **405** for Pablo Rodriguez's chart.
- Click on the **History and Physical** tab.

1. What electrolyte imbalances did Pablo Rodriguez present with on admission?

→ • Click on **Laboratory Reports**.

2. What was Pablo Rodriguez's calcium level on admission to the ED on Tuesday evening?

3. How does this level correlate with the physician's diagnosis? Speculate as to the reason for the discrepancy.

4. What was Pablo Rodriguez's phosphorous level during the same time frame?

5. How does this relate to his calcium level?

→ • Click on **History and Physical**.

6. What would be the most likely cause for hypercalcemia in this patient?

→ • Click on **Physician's Orders**.

7. What medication did the ED physician order to treat the hypercalcemia?

→ • Click on **Return to Nurses' Station**. Then click on either the **Drug Guide** on the counter or the **Drug** icon in the bottom left corner of your screen.

8. Describe the mechanism of action and therapeutic effect of the medication you identified in question 7.

9. What nursing assessments are appropriate related to the administration of this medication?

→ • Click on **Return to Nurses' Station**.
  • Click on **Chart** and then on **405**.
  • Click on **Laboratory Reports**.

10. What were Pablo Rodriguez's calcium and phosphorous levels this morning (Wednesday at 0730)?

11. Was the prescribed medication effective? Is the patient out of danger?

→ • Click on **Return to Nurses' Station**.
  • Click on **Kardex** and then on tab **405**.

12. What intravenous fluids is Pablo Rodriguez receiving?

13. What is the purpose of IV hydration in relation to serum calcium levels?

14. Is this the solution you would normally expect to administer to a patient with hypercalcemia? If not, what solution would you expect and why?

→ • Click on **Return to Nurses' Station**.
   • Click on **MAR** and then on tab **405**.

15. What medication is scheduled to be administered at 1500?

16. What electrolyte imbalance will this medication correct? Explain your answer. (*Hint:* Consult the Drug Guide in the Nurses' Station.)

17. What nursing assessments must be completed prior to administration of this drug?

18. Do you have any concerns regarding administering this drug at this specific time? (*Hint:* Review the patient's GI history on admission in the chart.)

→ • Click on **Return to Nurses' Station** and then on **405**.
   • Click on **Patient Care**.

19. Complete a physical assessment on Pablo Rodriguez (including vital signs). Document your findings below.

Areas Assessed	Findings on Physical Examination
Cardiovascular	
Respiratory	
Neuromuscular	
Gastrointestinal	

20. Is Pablo Rodriguez demonstrating any clinical manifestations of hypercalcemia? If yes, describe the pathophysiologic basis for the symptoms. If not, explain why not.

21. If Pablo Rodriguez had a calcium level of 13.5, what other clinical manifestations might you expect to find? (*Hint:* See page 240 in the textbook.)

22. When evaluating Pablo Rodriguez's renal output, what potential complication of hypercalcemia would you be alert for?

23. After successful treatment of Pablo Rodriguez, the nurse must be alert for overcorrecting of the electrolyte imbalance. For what clinical manifestations should the nurse monitor this patient related to hypocalcemia and hyperphosphatemia?

Acid-Base Imbalance

 Reading Assignment: Acid-Base Imbalance (Chapter 15)

Patients: Jacqueline Catanazaro, Room 402
Patricia Newman, Room 406

Goal: Utilize the nursing process to competently care for patients with acid-base imbalances.

Objectives:

1. Describe the pathophysiologic basis of acid-base imbalance noted in assigned patients.
2. Identify specific etiologic factor(s) related to respiratory acidosis in the assigned patients.
3. Assess the assigned patients for clinical manifestations related to respiratory acidosis.
4. Describe nursing interventions appropriate when caring for specific patients with respiratory acidosis.
5. Evaluate the effectiveness of medication prescribed to treat acid-base imbalances.

In this lesson you will assess, plan, and implement care for patients with acid-base imbalance. Jacqueline Catanazaro is a 45-year-old female admitted with excerabation of asthma and schizophrenia. Patricia Newman is a 61-year-old female admitted with pneumonia and a history of emphysema for 12 years. Begin this lesson by reviewing the general concepts of acid-base balance as presented in your textbook.

Exercise 1

 Clinical Preparation: Writing Activity

20 minutes

1. Define the following terms.

   a. pH

   b. Normal serum pH

   c. Neutral pH

   d. Acidic solution

   e. Alkaline solution

2. Identify and describe the three physiologic systems that work to maintain acid-basis home-ostasis by completing the following table.

System	Mechanisms of Action	Acid-Base Compensation
a.		
b.		
c.		

Exercise 2

 CD-ROM Activity

 45 minutes

- Sign in to work at Pacific View Regional Hospital for Period of Care 1. (*Note:* If you are already in the virtual hospital from a previous exercise, click on **Leave the Floor** and then **Restart the Program** to get to the sign-in window.)
- From the Patient List, select Jacqueline Catanazaro (Room 402).
- Click on **Go to Nurses' Station**.
- Click on **Chart** and then on **402**.
- Click on **History and Physical**.

1. Is there anything in Jacqueline Catanazaro's history that would put her at risk for an acid-base balance? Explain.

- Click on **Return to Nurses' Station** and then on **402**.
- Click on **Patient Care**.
- Click on **Nurse-Client Interaction**.
- Select and view the video titled **0730: Intervention—Airway**. (*Note:* If this video is not available, check the virtual clock to see whether enough time has elapsed. The video cannot be viewed before its specified time.)

2. Based on Jacqueline Catanazaro's history, what would you expect to be causing her respiratory distress?

3. Why is the nurse waiting until after the ABGs are drawn to give the patient a nebulizer treatment?

- Click on **Chart** and then on **402**.
- Click on **Laboratory Reports**.

4. What are the results of Jacqueline Catanazaro's two most recent ABGs? Document these results in the table below.

Results	Monday 1030	Wednesday 0730
pH		
PaO$_2$		
PaCO$_2$		
O$_2$ sat		
Bicarb		

5. How would you interpret the above results? Is the acid-base imbalance compensated or uncompensated (fully or partially)? Explain your answer.

6. Based on the acute aspect of Jacqueline Catanazaro's respiratory difficulties, what mechanism(s) would you expect to be working to compensate for her respiratory acidosis?

 7. If the patient had electrolyte results available, what might you expect her potassium levels to be? Explain your answer. (*Hint:* See page 250 in the textbook.)

8. Based on Jacqueline Catanazaro's medical diagnosis, what is the underlying pathophysiological problem leading to the respiratory acidosis? (*Hint:* See page 1808 of the textbook.)

→ • Click on **Return to Room 402**.

• Inside the patient's room, click on **Patient Care**.

9. Perform a complete physical assessment on Jacqueline Catanazaro and complete the table below.

Areas Assessed	Findings on Physical Examination
Neurologic	
Musculoskeletal	
Cardiovascular	
Respiratory	
Integumentary	

10. Are there any clinical manifestations of respiratory acidosis? Is so, please describe. If not, how do you explain this?

11. If Jacqueline Catanazaro had a pH level of 7.2, how might this assessment differ?

→ • Click on **Chart** and then on **402**.
  • Click on **Physician's Orders**.

12. Look at the most recent physician's orders. What medication is ordered to treat the patient's respiratory acidosis? What is the medication's underlying mechanism of action to correct the acidosis?

→ • Click on **Return to Room 402**.
  • Click on **Leave the Floor**.
  • Click on **Restart the Program**.
  • Log in to Period of Care 2 and select Jacqueline Catanazaro as your patient.
  • Click on **Go to Nurses' Station**.
  • Click on **Chart** and then on **402**.
  • Click on **Laboratory Reports**.

13. Look at the ABGs drawn at 1000. Interpret these results. Was the treatment effective?

Exercise 3

 CD-ROM Activity

 45 minutes

- Sign in to work at Pacific View Regional Hospital for Period of Care 1. (*Note:* If you are already in the virtual hospital from a previous exercise, click on **Leave the Floor** and then **Restart the Program** to get to the sign-in window.)
- From the Patient List, select Patricia Newman (Room 406).
- Click on **Nurses' Station**.
- Click on **Chart** and then on **406**.
- Click on **History and Physical**.

1. Is there anything in Patricia Newman's history that would put her at risk for an acid-base balance? Explain.

- Click on **Laboratory Reports**.

2. What are the results of Patricia Newman's two most recent ABGs? Document your findings below.

Results	Tuesday 2300	Wednesday 0500
pH		
PaO_2		
$PaCO_2$		
O_2 sat		
Bicarb		

3. How would you interpret the above results? Is the acid-base imbalance compensated or uncompensated (fully or partially)? Explain your answer.

4. Based on the chronic aspect of Patricia Newman's respiratory difficulties, what physiologic systems would you expect to be working to compensate for the respiratory acidosis?

5. Based on the ABG results, has Patricia Newman's condition improved or worsened since admission the evening before?

→ • While still in the Chart, click on **Nurse's Notes**.

6. Read the notes for Wednesday 0730. Describe the actions taken by the nurse. Are they appropriate or not? Explain you answer.

7. What additional actions do you think would be appropriate at this time?

→ • Click on **Laboratory Reports**.

8. What is the patient's serum potassium level?

9. How would you explain the patient's hypokalemia in concert with respiratory acidosis? (*Hint:* Check her concurrent medications and see page 250 in the textbook.)

 10. Based on Patricia Newman's medical diagnosis, what is the underlying pathophysiologic problem leading to the respiratory acidosis? (*Hint:* See page 1818 of the textbook). How does that differ from Jacqueline Catanazaro's problem in Exercise 2?

 • Click on **Return to Nurses' Station** and then on **406**.
• Click on **Patient Care**.

11. Perform a complete physical assessment, including vital signs, on Patricia Newman and complete the table below and on the next page.

Areas Assessed	Findings on Physical Examination
Neurologic	
Musculoskeletal	

Areas Assessed	Findings on Physical Examination
Cardiovascular	
Respiratory	
Integumentary	

12. Does Patricia Newman have any clinical manifestations of respiratory acidosis? Is so, please describe. If not, explain why not.

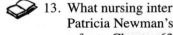 13. What nursing interventions could you, as a graduate nurse, plan and implement to improve Patricia Newman's acid-base balance and prevent complications? (*Hint:* You may need to refer to Chapter 63 in your textbook, which discusses the underlying cause of Patricia Newman's respiratory acidosis.)

Patients Having Surgery

 Reading Assignment: Clients Having Surgery (Chapter 16)

Patients: Piya Jordan, Room 403
Clarence Hughes, Room 404

Goal: Utilize the nursing process to competently care for perioperative patients.

Objectives:

1. Document a complete history and physical on a preoperative patient.
2. Identify appropriate rationale for preoperative orders on an assigned patient.
3. Evaluate completeness of preoperative teaching on a patient scheduled for surgery.
4. Document a focused assessment on a patient transferred from PACU to a medical-surgical unit.
5. Plan appropriate interventions to prevent postoperative complications in an assigned patient.
6. Utilize the nursing process to correctly administered scheduled and prn medications to an assigned patient.

In this lesson you will learn the essentials of caring for patients in both the preoperative and postoperative stages of surgery. You will document assessments, plan, implement, and evaluate care given. Piya Jordan is a 68-year-old female admitted with nausea and vomiting for 3 days. Clarence Hughes is a 73-year-old male admitted for an elective knee replacement.

Exercise 1

 CD-ROM Activity

40 minutes

- Sign in to work at Pacific View Regional Hospital for Period of Care 1. (*Note:* If you are already in the virtual hospital from a previous exercise, click on **Leave the Floor** and then **Restart the Program** to get to the sign-in window.)
- From the Patient List, select Piya Jordan (Room 403).
- Click on **Go to Nurses' Station**.
- Click on **Chart** and then on **403**.
- Click on **Emergency Department** and review this record.

1. What day and time did Piya Jordan arrive in the Emergency Department?

2. What complaints (problems) brought her to the ED?

3. What were Piya Jordan's primary and secondary admitting diagnoses?

→ • Click on **Nursing Admission**.

4. Important areas of data collection for the health history during the preoperative period are listed below and on the next page. Using the Nursing Admission form as your source, record the data collected for each area. If an area was not completed, write "No Data" in that section. (*Hint:* Refer to pages 264-266 of textbook for clarification of each section.)

Areas of Data Collection	Piya Jordan's Data
Previous surgery and experience with anesthesia	
Serious illness or trauma (ABCDE mnemonic)	
Alcohol, recreational drug, or nicotine use	
Current discomforts	
Chronic illnesses	
Advanced age	

Areas of Data Collection	Piya Jordan's Data
Medication history	
Psychologic history	
Ability to tolerate perioperative stress	
Lifestyle habits	
Social history	

➔ • Click on **History and Physical**.

5. In addition to data obtained from the health history, a physical examination provides necessary data for the preoperative assessment. For each of the areas listed below and on the next page, identify (in the middle column) the key items to assess according to your textbook (pages 266-272). In the last column, document the results from the physician's assessment as noted in the H&P. If an area was not completed, write "No Data" in that section. (*Note:* Do not include diagnostic testing; this will be addressed separately.)

Physical Examination Area	Key Specific Assessments from Textbook	Results for Piya Jordan
Cardiovascular		
Respiratory		

Physical Examination Area	Key Specific Assessments from Textbook	Results for Piya Jordan
Musculoskeletal		
Gastrointestinal		
Skin integrity		
Renal		
Cognitive and neurologic		

➡ • Click on **Laboratory Reports**.

6. The most common preoperative lab tests are listed in the chart below and on the next page. For each test, record results for Piya Jordan. If a test was not completed, write "No data."

Laboratory Tests	Piya Jordan's Results
Potassium	
Sodium	
Chloride	
Calcium	
Glucose (fasting)	
Carbon dioxide	

Laboratory Tests	**Piya Jordan's Results**
Creatinine	
BUN	
Albumin	
Prealbumin	
Hemoglobin	
Hematocrit	
WBC	
Differential Count	
Segmented neutrophils	
Banded neutrophils	
Eosinophils	
Basophils	
Lymphocytes	
Monocytes	
PT	
aPTT	

7. Are any of Piya Jordan's lab results abnormal or of concern for a patient preparing to undergo surgery? Explain.

8. Based on your findings during this exercise, how would you rate Piya Jordan's general surgical risk according to the American Society of Anesthesia? (*Hint:* See Box 16-3 in your textbook.)

Exercise 2

 CD-ROM Activity

 30 minutes

- Sign in to work at Pacific View Regional Hospital for Period of Care 1. (*Note:* If you are already in the virtual hospital from a previous exercise, click on **Leave the Floor** and then **Restart the Program** to get to the sign-in window.)
- From the Patient List, select Piya Jordan (Room 403).
- Click on **Go to Nurses' Station**.
- Click on **Chart** and then on **403**.
- Click on **Consents**.

1. For what procedure(s) has Piya Jordan given written consent?

2. Who signed the consent form as the witness?

3. Who is responsible for providing detailed information about the procedure(s) for which Piya Jordan has given consent?

4. What is the nurse's responsibility in regard to obtaining informed consent?

→ • Click on **Physician's Orders**.

5. Look at the orders for Tuesday 0130. What consent was ordered by the physician?

6. By when does this consent need to be obtained?

7. What is the purpose for the mineral oil enema that was ordered to be given to Piya Jordan?

8. What diet has the physician ordered preoperatively? What is the purpose for this diet order?

9. What is the rationale for giving Piya Jordan a unit of fresh frozen plasma preoperatively?

10. What is the rationale for ordering a dose of cefotetan on call to the OR? Is this a safe order to administer to Piya Jordan? Explain why or why not.

→ • Click on **Surgical Reports**.

11. Scroll down to the Preoperative Checklist. What preoperative teaching was completed?

12. The word "routines" on the preoperative checklist is not very explicit. Explain specific items that should have been taught to Piya Jordan preoperatively.

Exercise 3

 CD-ROM Activity

 45 minutes

You will now be reviewing immediate postoperative care as well as planning and evaluating care given during this time period.

- Sign in to work at Pacific View Regional Hospital for Period of Care 1. (*Note:* If you are already in the virtual hospital from a previous exercise, click on **Leave the Floor** and then **Restart the Program** to get to the sign-in window.)
- From the Patient List, select Clarence Hughes (Room 404).
- Click on **Go to Nurses' Station**.
- Click on **EPR** and then on **Login**.
- Select **404** from the Patient drop-down menu. Change categories as needed to answer question 1.

1. Upon arrival to the medical-surgical nursing unit, a postoperative patient requires an immediate focused assessment. Document the assessment findings recorded by the nurse on Sunday at 1600 when Clarence Hughes arrived on the unit according to the areas of focus noted below. (*Hint:* See textbook pages 305-309 for clarification of assessment areas.)

Focused Assessment Areas	Clarence Hughes' Assessment Findings
Respiratory status	
Circulatory status	
Neurologic status	
Wound status	
Intravenous fluids	

Focused Assessment Areas	**Clarence Hughes' Assessment Findings**

Drainage tubes

Pain

 2. How frequently did the nurse assess Clarence Hughes' vital signs after arrival on the unit? How often do you think they should be assessed? (*Hint:* See page 305 in your textbook.)

➔ • Still in the EPR, change the category to **Intake and Output**.

3. Review Clarence Hughes' I&O for the past 3 days. Document your findings below.

	Sun 1500-2300	Mon 2300-0700	Mon 0700-1500	Mon 1500-2300	Tues 2300-0700	Tues 0700-1500	Tues 1500-2300	Wed 2300-0700
Intake								
Output								

4. Which is greater—Clarence Hughes' intake or output? By how much? Is this expected?

5. What are the possible consequences if this trend in fluid balance continues?

→ • Click on **Exit EPR**.
• Click on **Chart** and then on **404**.
• Click on **Physician's Orders**.

6. Look at the physician's postoperative orders written on Sunday at 1600. What is ordered to prevent postoperative atelectasis and/or pneumonia?

7. What additional interventions could you, as the nurse, perform to further prevent atelectasis and/or pneumonia?

8. What is ordered to prevent DVT?

9. Scroll up to look at the orders for Monday 0715. What did the physician order at this time to prevent DVT postoperatively?

10. What additional intervention could you, as the nurse, perform to further prevent DVT?

11. If you were caring for Clarence Hughes postoperatively on Sunday, what incisional wound care would you perform?

• Click on **Return to Nurses' Station** and then on **404**.

• Once inside the patient's room, click on **Take Vital Signs**.

• After reviewing the patient's vital signs, click on **Clinical Alerts**.

• Next, click on **Patient Care** and then on **Nurse-Client Interactions**.

• Select and view the video titled **0735: Empathy**. (*Note:* If this video is not available, check the virtual clock to see whether enough time has elapsed. The video cannot be viewed before its specified time.)

12. What is Clarence Hughes' major concern at this point?

Medication Preparation

 • Click on **Medication Room** at the bottom of your screen.

• From the Medication Room, click on **MAR** to determine medications that Clarence Hughes is ordered to receive at 0800 and any appropriate prn medications you may want to administer. (*Note:* You may click on **Review MAR** at any time to verify correct medication order. Remember to look at the patient name on the MAR to make sure you have the correct patient's record—you must click on the correct room number within the MAR. Click on **Return to Medication Room** after reviewing the correct MAR.)

• Click on **Unit Dosage** at the top of your screen or on the Unit Dosage cabinet to the right of Automated System.

• From the close-up view of the Unit Dosage drawers, click on drawer **404**.

• From the list of available medications in the top window, select the medication(s) you would like to administer. After each medication you select, click on **Put Medication on Tray**.

• When you have finished putting your selected medications on the tray, click on **Close Drawer**.

• Click on **View Medication Room**.

• Next, click on **Automated System** (or on the Automated System unit itself). Your name and password will automatically appear. Click on **Login**.

• In box 1, select the correct patient; in box 2, choose the appropriate Automated System Drawer for this patient. Then click on **Open Drawer**.

• From the list of available medications, select the medication(s) you would like to administer. For each one selected, click on **Put Medication on Tray**. When you are finished, click on **Close Drawer**.

• Click **View Medication Room**.

• From the Medication Room, click on **Preparation** (or on the preparation tray on the counter); then highlight the medication you want to administer. Click on **Prepare**.

• Wait for the Preparation Wizard to appear; then provide any information requested.

• Click **Next**, choose the correct patient to administer this medication to, and click **Finish**.

• Repeat the previous two steps until you have prepared all the medications you want to administer.

• You can click **Review Your Medications** and then **Return to Medication Room** when you are ready. Once you are back in the Medication Room, you may go directly to Clarence Hughes' room by clicking on **404** at bottom of screen.

Medication Administration

 • Administer the medication, utilizing the five rights of medication administration. After you have collected the appropriate assessment data and are ready for administration, click **Patient Care** and then **Medication Administration**. Verify that the correct patient and medication(s) appear in the left-hand window. Then click the down arrow next to Select. From the drop-down menu, select **Administer** and complete the Administration Wizard by providing any information requested. When the Wizard stops asking for information, click **Administer to Patient**. Specify **Yes** when asked whether this administration should be recorded in the MAR. Finally, click **Finish**.

Now let's see how you did!

 • Click on **Leave the Floor** at the bottom of your screen. From the Floor Menu, select **Look at Your Preceptor's Evaluation**. Then click on **Medication Scorecard**.

13. Note below whether or not you correctly administered the appropriate medications. If not, why do you think you were incorrect? According to Table C in this scorecard, what are the appropriate resources that should be used and important assessments that should be completed prior to administering these medications? Did you use these resources and perform these assessments correctly?

LESSON **7**

Cancer

/OPO **Reading Assignment:** Perspectives in Oncology (Chapter 18)
Clients with Cancer (Chapter 19)
Management of Clients with Parenchymal and Pleural Disorders
(Chapter 64, pages 1852-1855)

Patient: Pablo Rodriguez, Room 405

Goal: Utilize the nursing process to competently care for patients with cancer.

Objectives:

1. Describe clinical manifestations and treatment for a patient with cancer.
2. Recognize special needs of patients undergoing treatment for cancer.
3. Appropriately treat a patient's symptoms related to disease process and/or side effects of treatment.
4. Discuss medications prescribed for a patient with cancer, including expected therapeutic effects as well as adverse/side effects to monitor for.
5. Plan appropriate general interventions to prevent and/or treat complications related to chemotherapy.

In this lesson you will learn the essentials of caring for a patient diagnosed with cancer. You will collect data, assess, plan, implement, and evaluate care given. Pablo Rodriguez is a 71-year-old male admitted with advanced lung carcinoma. Begin this lesson by reviewing the general concepts of cancer as presented in your textbook.

Exercise 1

 Clinical Preparation: Writing Activity

 20 minutes

1. Identify and briefly describe four types of carcinogens.

2. What are the three types of therapies used to treat cancer? Describe their respective mechanisms of action.

3. List common side effects of chemotherapy.

4. What are some common side effects associated with radiation therapy?

 5. List the warning signals associated with lung cancer (*Hint:* See Box 64-2 in your textbook.)

Exercise 2

 CD-ROM Activity

 35 minutes

- Sign in to work at Pacific View Regional Hospital for Period of Care 1. (*Note:* If you are already in the virtual hospital from a previous exercise, click on **Leave the Floor** and then **Restart the Program** to get to the sign-in window.)
- From the Patient List, select Pablo Rodriguez (Room 405).
- Click on **Go to Nurses' Station**.
- Click on **Chart** and then on **405**.
- Click on **History and Physical**.

1. What is Pablo Rodriguez's main diagnosis?

2. How long ago was he diagnosed?

3. What risk factor for lung cancer is documented on the H&P?

4. What are other risk factors for lung cancer? (*Hint:* See pages 613-614 of your textbook.)

5. What clinical manifestations documented in the physician's review of systems are related to this disease process?

6. What treatment has Pablo Rodriguez received so far?

7. How long ago did he receive his last chemotherapy?

8. What are the mechanism of action and the major side effects of docetaxel? (*Hint:* For help, return to the Nurses' Station and click on **Drug Guide** on the counter.)

9. What is the nadir (the point at which the drug has the greatest impact on the bone marrow) of docetaxel? Would the patient still be having side effects from this drug? Why or why not?

10. What interventions would you teach Pablo Rodriguez to prevent complications related to bone marrow suppression caused by chemotherapy?

Exercise 3

 CD-ROM Activity

 30 minutes

- Sign in to work at Pacific View Regional Hospital for Period of Care 2. (*Note:* If you are already in the virtual hospital from a previous exercise, click on **Leave the Floor** and then **Restart the Program** to get to the sign-in window.)
- From the Patient List, select Pablo Rodriguez (Room 405).
- Click on **Go to Nurses' Station**.
- Click on **Get Report** and read the change-of-shift report.

1. What unresolved problem for Pablo Rodriguez is noted in the change-of-shift report?

 • Click on **Go to Nurses' Station**.
- Click on **405** to go to Pablo Rodriguez's room.
- Click on **Chart** and then on **405**.
- Click on **Nurse's Notes**.

2. Look at the note for Wednesday at 0415. How did the nurse respond to Pablo Rodriguez's complaints? Were the nurse's actions appropriate? Explain.

3. How might you have responded differently?

 • Click on **Return to Nurses' Station**.
• Click on **405** to go to the patient's room.
• Inside the room, click on **Patient Care** and then on **Nurse-Client Interactions**.
• Select and view the video titled **0735: Patient Perceptions**. (*Note:* If this video is not available, check the virtual clock to see whether enough time has elapsed. The video cannot be viewed before its specified time.)

4. What are Pablo Rodriguez's two major concerns at this point?

5. What other assessment should you perform before treating his complaint of nausea?

 • Click on **MAR**.
• Click on tab **405** for Pablo Rodriguez's record.

6. What medications are ordered to manage the patient's pain and nausea?

7. What might the nurse question regarding these medication orders?

→ • Click on **Return to Room 405**.
  • Click on **Chart** and then on **405** for correct patient chart.
  • Click on **Nursing Admission**.

8. What is the patient's weight in pounds? In kgs?

→ • Click on **Return to Room 405**.
  • Click on the **Drug** icon in the lower left corner of your screen.

9. Calculate the maximum 24-hour dose for patients receiving the drug ordered for nausea related to chemotherapy.

10. Calculate the maximum 24-hour dose for management of postoperative nausea and vomiting.

11. Calculate the maximum amount of this drug Pablo Rodriguez could receive per 24 hours as ordered. Is it within the dosage guidelines? Is there any reason to be concerned about this dosage schedule over long periods of time?

12. What are the possible ramifications of giving high doses of this drug?

13. What are the ramifications of *not* giving this drug for the patient's complaint of nausea?

14. If the nurse administers the prn Reglan at 0730, what should be done with the regularly scheduled 0800 dose?

Exercise 4

 CD-ROM Activity

 40 minutes

- Sign in to work at Pacific View Regional Hospital for Period of Care 2. (*Note:* If you are already in the virtual hospital from a previous exercise, click on **Leave the Floor** and then **Restart the Program** to get to the sign-in window.)
- From the Patient List, select Pablo Rodriguez (Room 405).
- Click on **Go to Nurses' Station**.
- Click on **MAR** and then on **405** for Pablo Rodriguez's record.

1. What medications still need to be given to Pablo Rodriguez for the day shift (up to 1500)?

 • Click on **Return to Nurses' Station**.
- Use the Drug Guide to answer the next three questions. To access this resource, you can click on the **Drug Guide** on the counter or click on the **Drug** icon in the lower left corner of your screen.

2. How does ondansetron differ from metoclopramide in regard to antiemetic mechanism of action?

3. How fast would you infuse the IV ondansetron?

4. What is the expected benefit that Pablo Rodriguez will receive from dexamethasone? Over what time period should it be administered?

→ • Click on **Return to Nurses' Station**.
  • Click on **Chart** and then on **405** to access Pablo Rodriguez's chart.
  • Click on the **Patient Education** tab.

5. Has any teaching yet been completed? In your opinion, what is a priority and thus should have been completed on admission?

→ • Click on **Return to Nurses' Station** and then on **405** to go to the patient's room.
  • Click on **Patient Care**.
  • Click on **Nurse-Client Interactions**.
  • Select and view the video titled **1150: Assessment—Pain**. (*Note:* If this video is not available, check the virtual clock to see whether enough time has elapsed. The video cannot be viewed before its specified time.)

6. Why is the patient not eating?

7. Is this a normal side effect of chemotherapy?

8. How would you treat this?

→ • Click on **Kardex** and read the outcomes.

9. What additional outcome(s) might you include for this patient?

10. What is the patient's code status? How do you feel about this in relation to his diagnosis and condition? What is the nurse's professional responsibility related to the patient's code status?

LESSON **8** _____

Pain

_____

/○乃 **Reading Assignment:** Clients with Pain (Chapter 22)

Patients: Clarence Hughes, Room 404
Pablo Rodriguez, Room 405

Goal: Demonstrate understanding and application of appropriate interventions when caring for patients with pain.

Objectives:

1. Define the concept of pain.
2. Describe the source and type of pain for each patient.
3. Perform a comprehensive pain assessment for each patient.
4. Identify variables that influence each patient's perception of pain.
5. Safely administer analgesic medications to a patient experiencing pain.
6. Plan appropriate nonpharmacologic measures that may be used to treat each patient's pain.

In this lesson you will evaluate the pain experience of two different patients—from assessment to management. Clarence Hughes is a 73-year-old male who is status post total knee arthroplasty. Pablo Rodriguez is a 71-year-old male admitted with advanced lung carcinoma. Begin this activity by reviewing the general concepts presented in your textbook. Answer the following questions to solidify your understanding of pain.

Exercise 1

 Clinical Preparation: Writing Activity

 15 minutes

1. Using the definitions of pain provided in the textbook, describe pain in your own words.

2. What is the difference between a patient's pain threshold and pain tolerance?

3. What are the five key elements to the pain management standards of the Joint Commission on Accreditation of Healthcare Organizations (JCAHO)?

4. How do the American Pain Society's standards for pain management differ from those of JCACHO?

Exercise 2

 CD-ROM Activity

 45 minutes

- Sign in to work at Pacific View Regional Hospital for Period of Care 1. (*Note:* If you are already in the virtual hospital from a previous exercise, click on **Leave the Floor** and then **Restart the Program** to get to the sign-in window.)
- From the Patient List, select Clarence Hughes (Room 404).
- Click on **Get Report**.

1. What information is obtained during report concerning Clarence Hughes most recent pain assessment?

Now complete your own pain assessment on Clarence Hughes.

 • Click on **Go to Nurses' Station**.
- Click on **404** to go to the patient's room.
- Inside the room, click on **Take Vital Signs**.

2. How does Clarence Hughes rate his pain at the present time?

 • Click on **Patient Care**. Select the various body area buttons and assessment subcategories as needed to answer question 3.

3. Perform a focused assessment on Clarence Hughes. Record your findings below.

• Click on **Nurse-Client Interactions**.
  • Select and view the video titled **0730: Assessment/Perception of Care**. (*Note:* If this video is not available, check the virtual clock to see whether enough time has elapsed. The video cannot be viewed before its specified time.)

4. How does Clarence Hughes describe his pain? Describe his nonverbal communication. Do his nonverbal cues correlate with his complaint of pain?

5. The nurse asks Clarence Hughes if she may first perform an assessment prior to medicating him for pain. Is this appropriate? Why or why not?

 • Click on **EPR** and then on **Login**.
  • Select **404** for the patient's room and **Vital Signs** as the category.

6. Document Clarence Hughes' pain rating and characteristics over the last 24 hours in the table below and on the next page. (*Note:* You will complete the table in question 7.)

Time of Assessment	Pain Rating	Pain Characteristic	Name of Analgesic Administered
Tuesday 0700			
Tuesday 0815			
Tuesday 0930			
Tuesday 1230			
Tuesday 1330			
Tuesday 1500			
Tuesday 1630			
Tuesday 1700			
Tuesday 2030			

Time of Assessment	Pain Rating	Pain Characteristic	Name of Analgesic Administered
Tuesday 2300			
Wednesday 0200			
Wednesday 0715			

→ • Click on **Exit EPR**.
   • Click on **Chart** and then on **404**.
   • Click on **Expired MARs**.

7. Review the expired MARs to note the times of analgesic administration. Document your findings in the table in question 6.

→ • Click on **Return to Room 404**.
   • Click on **Kardex** and then on tab **404**.

8. What is the stated outcome related to comfort for Clarence Hughes? Is this a measurable outcome? How might you improve on the writing of the outcome?

9. In reviewing the table you completed for questions 6 and 7, was the administered pain medication effective? Explain your answer.

10. Was the patient's pain assessed appropriately following each analgesic administration? Explain your answer.

11. What is the physiologic source of Clarence Hughes' pain? What type of pain is he experiencing? Explain your answer. (*Hint:* See pages 447-448 of your textbook.)

12. Is the ordered analgesic medication appropriate for this type of pain? If not, what would you suggest? Are there any nonpharmacologic interventions that might be helpful for Clarence Hughes? Explain your answer.

13. What nursing assessments should be completed before administration of oxycodone with acetaminophen?

14. For what common side effects should the nurse monitor Clarence Hughes related to opioid use? (*Hint:* If you need help, return to the Nurses' Station and click on the **Drug Guide** on the counter or on the **Drug** icon in the lower left corner of your screen.)

- Click on **Return to Nurses' Station** (if not already there).
- Click on **Chart.**
- Click on **404** for Clarence Hughes' chart.
- Click on the **Nurse's Notes** tab and review the notes.

15. According to the note for Wednesday at 0715, which of the side effects identified in question 14 is Clarence Hughes experiencing? What should the nurse do to treat and/or prevent this side effect?

Since Clarence Hughes received his last dose of pain medication at 0200, it is now appropriate to administer another dose. Prepare to administer a dose of analgesic to Clarence Hughes by completing the following steps:

Medication Preparation

- Click on **Return to Nurses' Station**.
- Click on **Medication Room** on the bottom of your screen.
- Access the Automated System by either selecting the icon at the top of the screen or by clicking on the **Automated System** cart in center of screen.
- Click on **Login**.
- Choose Clarence Hughes in box 1 and Automated System Drawer (G-O) in box 2. Click **Open Drawer** and review the list of available medications. (*Note:* You may click **Review MAR** at any time to verify correct medication order. Remember to look at patient name on MAR to make sure you have the correct MAR—you must click on the correct room number within the MAR. Click on **Return to Medication Room** after reviewing the correct MAR.)
- From the Open Drawer view, select the correct medication to administer. Click **Put Medication on Tray** and then on **Close Drawer**.
- Click on **View Medication Room**.
- Begin the preparation process by clicking **Preparation** at the top of screen or clicking on the tray on the counter on the left side of the Medication Room.

- Click **Prepare**, fill in any requested data in the Preparation Wizard, and click **Next**. Then select the correct patient and click on **Finish**.
- You can click on **Review Your Medications** and then on **Return to Medication Room** when ready. Once you are back in the Medication Room, you may go directly to Clarence Hughes' room to administer this medication by clicking on **404** at the bottom of the screen.

Medication Administration

- Administer the medication utilizing five rights of medication administration. After you have collected the appropriate assessment data and are ready for administration, click **Patient Care** and then **Medication Administration**. Verify that the correct patient and medication(s) appear in the left-hand window. Then click the down arrow next to Select. From the drop-down menu, select **Administer** and complete the Administration Wizard by providing any information requested. When the Wizard stops asking for information, click **Administer to Patient**. Specify **Yes** when asked whether this administration should be recorded in the MAR. Finally, click **Finish**.

Now let's see how you did!

- Click on **Leave the Floor** at the bottom of your screen. From the Floor Menu, select **Look at Your Preceptor's Evaluation**. Then click on **Medication Scorecard**.

16. Disregard the report for the routine scheduled medications but note whether or not you correctly administered the analgesic medication. If not, why do you think you were incorrect in administering this drug? According to Table C in this scorecard, what are the appropriate resources that should be used prior to administering this medication? Did you use them correctly?

Exercise 3

 CD-ROM Activity

 45 minutes

- Sign in to work at Pacific View Regional Hospital for Period of Care 1. (*Note:* If you are already in the virtual hospital from a previous exercise, click on **Leave the Floor** and then **Restart the Program** to get to the sign-in window.)
- From the Patient List, select Pablo Rodriguez.
- Click on **Get Report**.

1. What information is obtained during report concerning Pablo Rodriguez's most recent pain assessment?

Now complete your own pain assessment of Pablo Rodriguez.

→ • Click on **Go to Nurses' Station**.
   • Click on **405**.
   • Click on **Take Vital Signs**.

2. How does Pablo Rodriguez rate his pain at the present time?

→ • Click on **Patient Care**.

3. Perform a focused assessment on Pablo Rodriguez. Document your findings below.

→ • Click on **Chart**.
   • Click on **405** for the correct patient chart.
   • Click on **Nursing Admission**.

4. Scroll down to page 22 of the Nursing Admission form. What are the aggravating and alleviating factors related to Pablo Rodriguez's pain?

- Click on **Return to Room 405** and then on **Patient Care**.
- Click on **Nurse-Client Interactions**.
- Select and view the video titled **0730: Symptom Management**. (*Note:* If this video is not available, check the virtual clock to see whether enough time has elapsed. The video cannot be viewed before its specified time.)

5. What sociocultural influences are affecting Pablo Rodriguez's perception and management of pain?

- Click on **EPR** and then on **Login**.
- Choose **405** for the patient's room and **Vital Signs** for the category.

6. Document Pablo Rodriguez's pain rating and characteristics since admission in the table below. (*Note:* You will complete this table in question 7.

Time of Assessment	Pain Rating	Pain Characteristic	Time of Medication Administration	Name of Analgesic Administered
Tuesday 2300				
			Wednesday 0100	
Wednesday 0300				
Wednesday 0700			Wednesday 0700	

- Click on **Exit EPR**.
- Click on **Chart** and then on **405**.
- Click on **Expired MARs**.

7. Review the expired MARs to find the times of analgesic administration. Document your findings under Name of Analgesic Administered in the table above.

• Click on **Return to Room 405**.

• Click on **Kardex**.

• Click on tab **405** for the correct record.

8. What is the stated outcome related to comfort for Pablo Rodriguez? Is this a measurable outcome? How might you improve on the writing of the outcome?

9. In reviewing the table you completed for questions 6 and 7 and your pain assessment in question 2, was the administered pain medication effective? Give a rationale for your answer.

10. Was the patient's pain assessed appropriately following each analgesic administration? Explain your answer.

11. What is the physiologic source of Pablo Rodriguez's pain? What type of pain is he experiencing? Explain your answer. (*Hint:* See pages 447-448 of your textbook.)

12. Is the ordered analgesic medication appropriate for this type of pain? If not, what would you suggest? Are there any nonpharmacologic interventions that might be helpful for Pablo Rodriguez? Explain your answer.

- Click on **Return to Room 405**.
- Click on **Nurse-Client Interactions**.
- Select and view the video titled **0735: Patient Perceptions**. (*Note:* If this video is not available, check the virtual clock to see whether enough time has elapsed. The video cannot be viewed before its specified time.)

13. Discuss the nurse's evaluation of Pablo Rodriguez's understanding and use of the PCA pump. Do you think the nurse's actions are therapeutic? If not, what other approaches would you suggest?

14. What nursing assessments and interventions are appropriate for patients receiving IV morphine sulfate? (*Note:* For help, return to the Nurses' Station and click on the **Drug Guide** on the counter or click on the **Drug** icon in the lower left corner of your screen.)

Palliative Care

 Reading Assignment: Perspectives in Palliative Care (Chapter 23)

Patient: Pablo Rodriguez, Room 405

Goal: Demonstrate understanding and appropriate application of palliative care concepts.

Objectives:

1. Identify appropriate application of palliative care concepts for a patient with a terminal illness.
2. Assess and identify common distressing symptoms present in a terminally ill patient.
3. Choose interventions appropriate to relieve distressing symptoms in a terminally ill patient.
4. Describe appropriate communication techniques when dealing with a terminally ill patient and family.

In this lesson you will describe, plan, and evaluate the care of a patient with a terminal illness that is no longer responding to therapy. Pablo Rodriguez is a 71-year-old male suffering from advanced lung carcinoma, diagnosed 1 year ago.

Exercise 1

Clinical Preparation: Writing Activity

10 minutes

1. Define *palliative care*.

2. Identify seven symptoms at the end of life that a palliative plan of care would address.

Exercise 2

 CD-ROM Activity

 30 minutes

- Sign in to work at Pacific View Regional Hospital for Period of Care 3. (*Note:* If you are already in the virtual hospital from a previous exercise, click on **Leave the Floor** and then **Restart the Program** to get to the sign-in window.)
- From the Patient List, select Pablo Rodriguez (Room 405).
- Click on **Go to Nurses' Station**.
- Click on **Chart** and then on **405**.
- Click on the **Emergency Department** tab.

1. Why was Pablo Rodriguez admitted to the hospital?

2. What are his primary and secondary diagnoses?

→ • Click on **Nursing Admission**.

3. What does the admitting nurse document for this patient's anticipated needs for support at time of discharge?

4. What documentation in the Nursing Admission would support the presence of cachexia-anorexia syndrome in Pablo Rodriguez?

5. What collaborative interventions would be appropriate to address Pablo Rodriguez's nutritional problems?

6. What distressing symptoms are noted in the Activity/Rest section of the Nursing Admission form?

7. What interventions would you plan for Pablo Rodriguez to alleviate these concerns?

 • Click on **Return to Nurses' Station** and then on **405**.
 • Click on **Patient Care**.
 • Click on **Nurse-Client Interactions**.
 • Select and view the video titled **1530: Decision—End-of-Life Care**. (*Note:* If this video is not available, check the virtual clock to see whether enough time has elapsed. The video cannot be viewed before its specified time.)

8. What is Pablo Rodriguez telling the nurse?

9. What therapeutic communication techniques is the nurse using? Are they effective? What other technique(s) might have been used?

 10. Although Pablo Rodriguez's family is not currently present, how might the nurse plan to help the family meet the patient's physical and emotional needs when he goes home? (*Hint:* See Table 23-7 in the textbook.)

Exercise 3

 CD-ROM Activity

 45 minutes

- Sign in to work at Pacific View Regional Hospital for Period of Care 1. (*Note:* If you are already in the virtual hospital from a previous exercise, click on **Leave the Floor** and then **Restart the Program** to get to the sign-in window.)
- From the Patient List, select Pablo Rodriguez (Room 405).
- Click on **Go to Nurses' Station**.
- Click on **405** to go to the patient's room.
- Read the Initial Observation at 0730.

1. According to the initial observation of Pablo Rodriguez, what physical symptom of distress is he displaying?

2. How would you intervene to alleviate Pablo Rodriguez's symptoms? Provide rationales for your interventions. (*Hint:* You made need to go to the patient's chart to review the physician's orders.)

 - Click on **EPR**.
- Click **Login**.
- Select **405** as the patient's room and **Vital Signs** as the category.
- Look at the vital sign assessment documented on Wednesday at 0700.

3. Describe Pablo Rodriguez's pain assessment.

4. What interventions would be appropriate to relieve this pain?

Now let's check the patient's current vital signs.

- Click on **Exit EPR**.
- Click on **Room 405** at the bottom of your screen.
- Click on **Take Vital Signs**. (Note that pain assessment is now considered the fifth vital sign.)

5. Based on the EPR data and Pablo Rodriguez's current pain rating, is the morphine providing effective relief? Explain.

- Click on **Patient Care**.
- From the list of body areas (the yellow buttons), click on **Abdomen**.
- From the system subcategories, click on **Gastrointestinal**.

6. Document your assessment findings below. What is this significance of these findings? How do they relate to Pablo Rodriguez's diagnosis and/or treatment?

7. How would you intervene to prevent potential complications related to the above findings?

• Click on **Nurse-Client Interactions**.
 • Select and view the video titled **0730: Symptom Management**. (*Note:* If this video is not available, check the virtual clock to see whether enough time has elapsed. The video cannot be viewed before its specified time.)

8. Describe Pablo Rodriguez's emotional distress as displayed in this video.

9. What nursing interventions would be appropriate to help Pablo Rodriguez cope?

 • Now select and view the video titled **0735: Patient Perceptions**.

10. Now that his pain is controlled, in addition to not being able to rest, what does Pablo Rodriguez complain of? How would you intervene to relieve this discomfort?

11. Recall the definition of palliative care. Based on your observations during this activity, do you believe Pablo Rodriguez is receiving such care? Why or why not?

Substance Abuse

Reading Assignment:
Clients with Substance Abuse Disorders (Chapter 26)

Patient: Harry George, Room 401

Goal: Demonstrate understanding and appropriate application of nursing interventions for patients with substance abuse.

Objectives:

1. Identify risk factors associated with substance abuse.
2. Describe assessment findings related to the use and abuse of nicotine and alcohol.
3. Describe assessment findings related to withdrawal from nicotine and alcohol.
4. Examine alcohol withdrawal protocols for the care of a patient admitted to an acute care setting.
5. Identify appropriate nursing interventions when caring for a patient with substance abuse.

In this lesson you will learn about the care of a patient undergoing specific substance abuse issues. Harry George is a 54-year-old male admitted with infection and swelling of his left foot and a history of type 2 diabetes. Begin this activity by reviewing the general concepts presented in your textbook. Answer the following questions to solidify your understanding of substance abuse.

Exercise 1

Clinical Preparation: Writing Activity

10 minutes

1. Define *substance abuse*.

2. What is the difference between physiologic and psychologic dependence?

3. Define the term *addiction*.

Exercise 2

 CD-ROM Activity

 30 minutes

- Sign in to work at Pacific View Regional Hospital for Period of Care 1. (*Note:* If you are already in the virtual hospital from a previous exercise, click on **Leave the Floor** and then **Restart the Program** to get to the sign-in window.)
- From the Patient List, select Harry George (Room 401).
- Click on **Go to Nurses' Station**.
- Click on **Chart** and then on **401**.
- Click on **Emergency Department** and read this record.

1. What are Harry George's primary and secondary diagnoses?

2. What specific risk factors for alcoholism are noted in the Emergency Department Record (*Hint:* Read the admitting physician notes.) Describe how the risk factors contribute to alcohol abuse.

3. When did Harry George begin drinking excessively? Was there a precipitating event that contributed to this problem?

4. What other documentation is found in the Emergency Department Record to support the diagnosis of alcohol abuse?

5. Is there any evidence of nicotine addiction?

➤ • Click on **History and Physical**.

6. Read the physical examination report on page 4. What assessment findings may be related to Harry George's alcohol abuse?

7. What further history is obtained regarding nicotine abuse?

8. What physical examination finding(s) may be related to cigarette smoking?

→ • Click on **Laboratory Reports**.

    9. What was Harry George's blood alcohol level on admission?

   10. What clinical manifestations would you expect to find based on this level?

→ • Click on **Return to Nurses' Station**.
  • Click on **401** to go to Harry George's room.
  • Click on **Patient Care**.
  • Click on **Nurse-Client Interactions**.
  • Select and view the video titled **0735: Symptom Management**. (*Note:* If this video is not available, check the virtual clock to see whether enough time has elapsed. The video cannot be viewed before its specified time.)

  11. What visual assessment findings noted on this video might suggest withdrawal symptoms for Harry George?

Exercise 3

 CD-ROM Activity

 45 minutes

- Sign in to work at Pacific View Regional Hospital for Period of Care 4. (*Note:* If you are already in the virtual hospital from a previous exercise, click on **Leave the Floor** and then **Restart the Program** to get to the sign-in window.)
- From the Patient List, select Harry George (Room 401).
- Click on **Go to Nurses' Station**.
- Click on **Chart** and then on **401**.
- Click on the **Mental Health** tab.

1. Read the Psychiatric/Mental Health Assessment for Harry George. What risk factors for substance abuses are noted on this assessment?

⟶ • Click on **Nurse's Notes**.

2. How does the nurse describe Harry George's behavior now?

 3. The textbook identifies the following symptoms of patients in alcohol withdrawal. Put an X next to all that apply for Harry George.

_____ a. Tremors

_____ b. Weakness

_____ c. Nausea

_____ d. Vomiting

_____ e. Sweating

_____ f. Tachycardia

_____ g. Hypertension

_____ h. Agitated behavior

_____ i. Delusions

_____ j. Hallucinations and nocturnal illusions

→ • Click on **History and Physical**.

4. At the end of the H&P, the physician writes a plan of care. What pharmacologic interventions is the physician planning to prevent and/or treat alcohol withdrawal?

5. What is the intended benefit of thiamine administration for this patient? (*Hint:* For help, return to the Nurses' Station and click on the **Drug Guide** on the counter or click on the **Drug** icon in the lower left corner of your screen.)

6. What is the classification of chlordiazepoxide? Identify this drug's most common brand name. What is the intended therapeutic effect of this drug for Harry George?

 7. What are the advantages of using medications in the above classification over other types of medications? (*Hint:* See page 545 of textbook of your textbook.)

 → • Click on **Nurse's Notes**. (*Note:* If you are currently within the Drug Guide, first click **Return to Nurses' Station**; then click on **Chart** and on **401**.)

8. Read the notes dated Wednesday at 1245 and at 1315. Is the chlordiazepoxide effective? Explain your answer.

9. What is the classification of lorazepam? Identify this drug's most common brand name. What is the intended therapeutic effect of this drug for Harry George?

10. Are there any potential drug interactions between chlordiazepoxide and lorazepam? Is so, please elaborate.

11. Since both Librium and Ativan are ordered for similar therapeutic effect, what factors would influence the nurse's decision regarding which medication to use? (*Hint:* Consult the MAR.)

→ • Click on **Physician's Orders**. (*Note:* If you are currently in the MAR, you must first **Return to Nurses' Station**; then click on **Chart** and **401**.)

12. What is the most recent physician order?

→ • Click on **Physician's Notes**.

13. Read the most recent physician's progress note. What is the rationale for writing the order you identified in question 12?

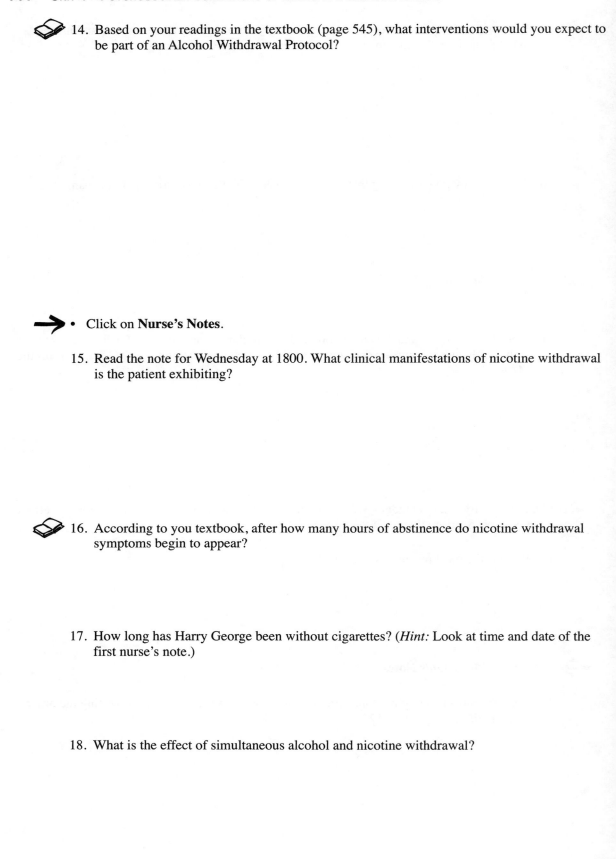

14. Based on your readings in the textbook (page 545), what interventions would you expect to be part of an Alcohol Withdrawal Protocol?

→ • Click on **Nurse's Notes**.

15. Read the note for Wednesday at 1800. What clinical manifestations of nicotine withdrawal is the patient exhibiting?

16. According to you textbook, after how many hours of abstinence do nicotine withdrawal symptoms begin to appear?

17. How long has Harry George been without cigarettes? (*Hint:* Look at time and date of the first nurse's note.)

18. What is the effect of simultaneous alcohol and nicotine withdrawal?

19. What typical manifestations of nicotine withdrawal might be found in another patient withdrawing *only* from nicotine?

20. To plan nursing care for Harry George, identify three priority nursing diagnoses for the patient problems listed in the table below. For each diagnosis, identify related patient outcomes and appropriate nursing interventions to achieve these outcomes.

Patient Problems (Assessment)	Nursing Diagnosis	Goals/Outcomes (Planning)	Nursing Interventions
Tremors			
Anxiety			
Malnutrition			

LESSON **11**

Osteoarthritis and Total Knee Replacement

Reading Assignment: Management of Clients with Musculoskeletal Disorders
(Chapter 28)

Patient: Clarence Hughes, Room 404

Goal: Utilize the nursing process to competently care for patients with musculoskeletal disorders.

Objectives:

1. Describe clinical manifestations and treatment for a patient with debilitating osteoarthritis.
2. Document a focused assessment on a postoperative patient who has undergone a total knee arthroplasty.
3. Plan appropriate interventions to prevent complications related to a total knee replacement in assigned patient.
4. Identify and provide rationale for collaborative care measures used to treat a patient after a total knee arthroplasty.

In this lesson you will learn the essentials of caring for a patient undergoing a total knee arthroplasty for treatment of debilitating osteoarthritis. You will document assessments, plan, implement, and evaluate care given. Clarence Hughes is a 73-year-old male admitted for an elective knee replacement. Begin this lesson by reviewing the general concepts of acid-base balance as presented in your textbook.

Exercise 1

 Clinical Preparation: Writing Activity

 10 minutes

1. Briefly describe the general pathophysiology of osteoarthritis (OA).

2. List risk factors related to the occurrence of primary OA.

3. What are the clinical manifestations of OA?

4. What laboratory and/or radiographic testing are used in the diagnosis of OA?

Exercise 2

 CD-ROM Activity

40 minutes

- Sign in to work at Pacific View Regional Hospital for Period of Care 1. (*Note:* If you are already in the virtual hospital from a previous exercise, click on **Leave the Floor** and then **Restart the Program** to get to the sign-in window.)
- From the Patient List, select Clarence Hughes (Room 404).
- Click on **Go to Nurses' Station**.
- Click on **Chart** and then on **404**.
- Click on **History and Physical**.

1. Why was Clarence Hughes admitted to the hospital?

2. Describe the symptoms that brought him to this point.

3. According to the H&P what medications and/or treatments were used to treat Clarence Hughes before he elected to have surgery?

4. Explain the rationale for performing a total knee replacement on Clarence Hughes.

- Click on **Surgical Reports**.

5. How does the report of operation describe the surgical procedure performed on Clarence Hughes?

6. Based on your reading from the textbook, what can you add to the description of a total knee arthroplasty?

7. What medication was added to the cement used for this procedure? Explain the rationale for the use of this medication.

8. What was Clarence Hughes' estimated blood loss (EBL)?

→ • Click on **Physician's Orders**.
  • Scroll down to read the orders for Sunday 1600.

9. What frequent assessments are ordered? Describe specifically how these assessments are completed and what the nurse is looking for.

10. What drain is ordered for Clarence Hughes? What is the expected amount of drainage?

- Click on **Return to Nurses' Station**.
- Click on **EPR** and then on **Login**.
- Select **404** for the patient's room.
- Choose **Intake and Output** as the category.

11. Find "Output: Drain #1" for documentation of hemovac drainage. How much total drainage is recorded?

- Click on **Exit EPR**.
- Then click on **Chart** and on **404** for Clarence Hughes' chart.
- Click on **Physician's Orders**.
- Find the orders for Monday 0715.

12. What is ordered to prevent knee contractures? Explain the basic use of this device.

13. According to your textbook (page 595), what does evidence-based practice conclude regarding the use of the CPM machine?

14. How should Clarence Hughes' operative leg be positioned at night? Explain the rationale for this position?

→ • Click on **Laboratory Reports**.

15. What was Clarence Hughes' H&H on Tuesday at 0600?

16. Why do you think his H&H was decreased? (*Hint:* Check his admitting H&H, EBL, drainage output, and intravenous intake.)

→ • Click on **Physician's Orders**.

17. What was ordered to correct the above laboratory result?

Exercise 3

 CD-ROM Activity

 45 minutes

- Sign in to work at Pacific View Regional Hospital for Period of Care 1. (*Note:* If you are already in the virtual hospital from a previous exercise, click on **Leave the Floor** and then **Restart the Program** to get to the sign-in window.)
- From the Patient List, select Clarence Hughes (Room 404).
- Click on **Get Report**.

1. What are your concerns for Clarence Hughes after receiving report?

→ • Click on **Go to Nurses' Station**.
   • Click on **404** to go to patient's room.
   • Click on **Patient Care**.

2. Based on Clarence Hughes' diagnosis and surgery, complete a focused assessment and document your findings below.

Area Assessed	Findings
Integumentary	
Musculoskeletal	
Neurovascular	
Gastrointestinal	
Respiratory	

• Click on **Clinical Alerts**.

   3. Based on these findings, what would be your priority interventions?

Medication Preparation

 • Click on **Medication Room**.

- Click on **MAR** to determine prn medications that have been ordered for Clarence Hughes to address his constipation and pain. (*Note:* You may click on **Review MAR** at any time to verify correct medication order. Remember to look at the patient name on the MAR to make sure you have the correct patient's record—you must click on the correct room number within the MAR. Click on **Return to Medication Room** after reviewing the correct MAR.)
- Click on **Unit Dosage** (or on the Unit Dosage cabinet); from the close-up view, click on drawer **404**.
- Select the medications you would like to administer. After each selection, click **Put Medication on Tray**. When you are finished selecting medications, click **Close Drawer**.
- Click on **View Medication Room**.
- Click on **Automated System** (or on the Automated System unit itself). Click **Login**.
- On the next screen, specify the correct patient and drawer location.
- Select the medication you would like to administer and click on **Put Medication on Tray**. Repeat this process if you wish to administer other medications from the Automated System.
- When you are finished, click **Close Drawer**. At the bottom right corner of the next screen, click on **View Medication Room**.
- From the Medication Room, click on **Preparation** (or on the preparation tray).
- From the list of medications on your tray, choose the correct medication to administer.
- Click **Next**, specify the correct patient to administer this medication to, and click **Finish**.
- Repeat the previous two steps until all medications that you want to administer are prepared.
- You can click on **Review Your Medications** and then on **Return to Medication Room** when ready. Once you are back in the Medication Room, you may go directly to Clarence Hughes' room by clicking on **404** at bottom of screen.

Medication Administration

 • Administer the medication, utilizing the five rights of medication administration. After you have collected the appropriate assessment data and are ready for administration, click **Patient Care** and then **Medication Administration**. Verify that the correct patient and medication(s) appear in the left-hand window. Then click the down arrow next to Select. From the drop-down menu, select **Administer** and complete the Administration Wizard by providing any information requested. When the Wizard stops asking for information, click **Administer to Patient**. Specify **Yes** when asked whether this administration should be recorded in the MAR. Finally, click **Finish**. You will evaluate your performance in this area at the end of this exercise (see question 14).

4. What is missing on the patient's order for oxycodone with acetaminophen? What measures need to be taken?

5. Based on the knowledge that most antacids decrease absorption of other medications when concurrently administered, what options might the nurse employ to ensure adequate absorption of pain medication? (*Hint:* To consult the Drug Guide, return to the Nurses' Station and click on the **Drug Guide** on the counter or click on the **Drug** icon in the lower left corner of your screen.)

→ • Click on **Nurse-Client Interactions**.
• Select and view the video titled **0735: Empathy**. (*Note:* If this video is not available, check the virtual clock to see whether enough time has elapsed. The video cannot be viewed before its specified time.)

6. In the video, the nurse attempts to appear empathetic by offering to listen to the patient's concerns. Are her actions congruent with her verbal communication? Why or why not?

7. What would you, as a student nurse, do differently?

8. Potential complications related to Clarence Hughes' postoperative status are listed below. While planning nursing care for this patient, identify measures that can be employed to pre-vent these complications. Document your plan of care below. (*Hint:* Postoperative care for a patient with a TKA is similar to care for a patient with a THA.)

Complications	Preventative Measures
Neurovascular compromise	
Wound infection	
Contractures/ Limited range of motion	
DVT	
Bleeding/anemia	

→ • Click on **Chart** and then on **404**.
  • Click on **Consultations**.

9. What is physical therapy (PT) doing for Clarence Hughes?

➤ • Click on **Physician's Orders**.

10. What is the patient's activity order for Wednesday morning?

➤ • Click on **Nurse's Notes**.

11. What is the patient's goal for CPM therapy today?

12. Do you think the ambulation and CPM goals are sufficient for the patient to be discharged tomorrow? Why or why not? (*Hint:* Review his home situation in the Nursing Admission form.)

➤ • Click on **Patient Education**.

13. What teaching should be completed for Clarence Hughes prior to discharge?

Now let's see how you did with the medication administration!

- Click on **Leave the Floor** at the bottom of your screen. From the Floor Menu, select **Look at Your Preceptor's Evaluation**. Then click on **Medication Scorecard**.

14. Ignore the report for the regularly scheduled medications. Note below whether or not you correctly administered the appropriate prn medications. If not, why do you think you were incorrect? According to Table C in this scorecard, what are the appropriate resources that should be used and important assessments that should be completed before administering these medications? Did you use these resources and perform these assessments correctly?

Osteoporosis

Reading Assignment: Management of Clients with Musculoskeletal Disorders (Chapter 28)

Patient: Patricia Newman, Room 406

Goal: Utilize the nursing process to competently care for patients with osteoporosis.

Objectives:

1. Describe the pathophysiology of osteoporosis.
2. Assess the patient for clinical manifestations of osteoporosis.
3. Describe appropriate pharmacologic therapy for prevention and/or treatment of osteoporosis.
4. Administer medications safely and accurately.
5. Plan appropriate interventions to promote health and prevent further bone loss in a patient with osteoporosis.
6. Develop an individualized teaching plan for an assigned patient with osteoporosis.

In this lesson you will learn the essentials of caring for a patient diagnosed with osteoporosis. You will explore the patient's history, evaluate presenting symptoms and treatment, administer prescribed medications, and develop an individualized discharge teaching plan. Patricia Newman is a 61-year-old female admitted with pneumonia and a history of emphysema.

Exercise 1

Clinical Preparation: Writing Activity

 20 minutes

1. Define the following terms.

    a. Bone mineral density (BMD or BMC)

b. T-score

c. Osteopenia

d. Osteoporosis

e. Severe (established) osteoporosis

f. Osteoclasts

g. Osteoblasts

2. What two factors determine a patient's risk of fragility fracture related to osteoporosis?

3. List the risk factors associated with osteoporosis.

Exercise 2

 CD-ROM Activity

 35 minutes

- Sign in to work at Pacific View Regional Hospital for Period of Care 2. (*Note:* If you are already in the virtual hospital from a previous exercise, click on **Leave the Floor** and then **Restart the Program** to get to the sign-in window.)
- From the Patient List, select Patricia Newman (Room 406).
- Click on **Go to Nurses' Station**
- Click on **Chart** and then on **406** for Patricia Newman's record.
- Click on **History and Physical**.

1. How long has Patricia Newman been diagnosed with osteoporosis?

2. What risk factors does Patricia Newman have for osteoporosis? Are any of these modifiable? If so, which ones?

3. What diagnostic test would have been ordered to diagnose Patricia Newman's osteoporosis? Describe the test and the result that would indicate osteoporosis.

→ • Click on **Laboratory Reports**.

4. Do any laboratory results for Patricia Newman correlate with osteoporosis?

5. What other laboratory result might you look at in relation to bone density?

→ • Click on **Nursing Admission**.

6. Are there any other risk factors found here? If so, what are they?

7. What clinical manifestation of osteoporosis is documented on this form?

8. For what other clinical manifestations would you assess Patricia Newman in relation to osteoporosis?

→ • Click on **Return to Nurses' Station**.
 • Click on **MAR** and then on **406** for Patricia Newman's record.

9. What medications are ordered for Patricia Newman to help treat and prevent worsening of her osteoporosis? Document the medications, their classification, and their respective mechanisms of action in the following table. You will complete the last column in question 10. (*Hint:* For help, return to the Nurses' Station and click on the **Drug Guide** on the counter or click on the **Drug** icon in the lower left corner of your screen.)

Medication	Drug Classification	Mechanism of Action	Side Effects

10. For what side effects should you monitor Patricia Newman related to these medications. Document your answer in the table above.

11. If you were to administer the prescribed estradiol to Patricia Newman, how and where would you apply this medication? Are there any precautions you should take while applying this?

Exercise 3

 CD-ROM Activity

 35 minutes

- Sign in to work at Pacific View Regional Hospital for Period of Care 3. (*Note:* If you are already in the virtual hospital from a previous exercise, click on **Leave the Floor** and then **Restart the Program** to get to the sign-in window.)
- From the Patient List, select Patricia Newman (Room 406).
- Click on **Go to Nurses' Station**.
- Click on **Chart** and then on **406**.
- Click on **Patient Education**.

1. What educational goals already identified could be related to Patricia Newman's osteoporosis?

2. What teaching would you provide Patricia Newman regarding exercise to prevent further bone loss? What types of exercises might benefit her?

3. What dietary needs does Patricia Newman have related to the osteoporosis? What foods would you teach her to include in her diet?

4. Complete the following chart to document teaching points you would you review with Patricia Newman regarding her medications to treat osteoporosis.

Medication	Teaching Points
Calcium carbonate 600 mg PO TID and at bedtime	

Estradiol 0.05 mg per 24 hours
  transdermal patch 2 times a week—
  Tuesday and Saturday	

5. If Patricia Newman asked you what further treatment might be available to her if her bone loss continued despite her present regimen, how would you answer her? (*Hint:* Identify four other drugs, or classifications of drugs, that might be useful to her and describe their mechanism of action.)

6. What is Patricia Newman most at risk for related to her osteoporosis?

7. What can you teach her that would help prevent this from occurring at home?

→ • Click on **Return to Nurses' Station** and then on **406** to go to the patient's room.
  • Click on **Patient Care**.
  • Click on **Nurse-Client Interactions**.
  • Select and view the video titled **1500: Discharge Planning**. (*Note:* If this video is not available, check the virtual clock to see whether enough time has elapsed. The video cannot be viewed before its specified time.)

8. Although the discussion in this video was related to Patricia Newman's pulmonary disease, how would smoking cessation benefit her musculoskeletal problem?

9. What other health care disciplines might be useful to help Patricia Newman with her discharge needs related to osteoporosis?

10. What psychosocial nursing diagnosis might be a potential problem for Patricia Newman related to her slightly stooped posture and going home on oxygen? What nursing interventions would be appropriate to help the patient with this difficulty?

LESSON 13 ────

Osteomyelitis and Wound Care

────────────────────

 Reading Assignment: Clients with Wounds (Chapter 20)

Management of Clients with Musculoskeletal Disorders (Chapter 28)

Patient: Harry George, Room 401

Goal: Utilize the nursing process to competently care for a patient with osteomyelitis and a chronic wound.

Objectives:

1. Assess an assigned patient for clinical manifestations of osteomyelitis.
2. Describe the causative agent and etiology of osteomyelitis in an assigned patient.
3. Safely administer IV antibiotic therapy as prescribed for osteomyelitis.
4. Evaluate diagnostic tests related to osteomyelitis.
5. Develop an appropriate plan of care for a patient with a chronic wound.
6. Develop an individualized discharge plan of care of a patient with osteomyelitis complicated by other disease processes and homelessness.

In this lesson you will learn the essentials of caring for a patient with an open wound who is also diagnosed with osteomyelitis. You will explore the patient's history, evaluate presenting symptoms and treatment, administer prescribed medications, and develop an individualized discharge teaching plan. Harry George is a 54-year-old male admitted with infection and swelling of his left foot, history of type 2 diabetes, alcohol abuse, and nicotine addiction.

Exercise 1

Clinical Preparation: Writing Activity

10 minutes

1. Identify risk factors for osteomyelitis.

2. What is the most common causative organism of osteomyelitis?

3. Identify and describe eight basic concepts of wound management.

Exercise 2

CD-ROM Activity

35 minutes

- Sign in to work at Pacific View Regional Hospital for Period of Care 2. (*Note:* If you are already in the virtual hospital from a previous exercise, click on **Leave the Floor** and then **Restart the Program** to get to the sign-in window.)
- From the Patient List, select Harry George (Room 401).
- Click on **Go to Nurses' Station**.
- Click on **Chart** and then on **401**.
- Click on **History and Physical**.

1. The clinical manifestations of osteomyelitis can include both local and systemic symptoms. Common local and systemic signs and symptoms are listed below. Place an X next to any signs or symptoms consistent with Harry George's history and his physical examination findings on admission.

_____ a. Acute localized pain	_____ g. Fever
_____ b. Swelling	_____ h. Night sweats
_____ c. Redness	_____ i. Nausea
_____ d. Drainage	_____ j. Malaise
_____ e. Warmth at infection site	_____ k. Chills
_____ f. Restricted movement	_____ l. Restlessness

2. Based on what you have read, identify the source (etiology) of Harry George's osteomyelitis. Explain the rationale for your conclusion.

3. What factors in Harry George's history may have contributed to the development of osteomyelitis?

→ • Click on **Physician's Orders**.

4. What diagnositic tests did the physician order to evaluate Harry George's osteomyelitis?

→ • Click on **Return to Nurses' Station**.
• Click on **MAR** and then on tab **401**.

5. Determine what routine medications (excluding the continuous IV and insulin coverage) you will be giving to Harry George during the day shift (0700-1500). Below, list the medications you need to give, the drug classification, the reason why each is given, and the time each is due. (*Hint:* For help, return to the Nurses' Station and click on the **Drug Guide** on the counter or click on the **Drug** icon in the bottom left corner of your screen.)

Medication	Classification	Reason for Giving	Time Due

6. Which medication was Harry George receiving that was discontinued on Tuesday?

→ • Click on **Return to Nurses' Station**.
  • Click on **Chart** and then on **401** for Harry George's record.
  • Click on **Physician's Orders**.

7. What replaced the medication you identified in question 6?

→ • Click on **Physician's Notes**.

8. Why was this change ordered?

→ • Click on **Laboratory Reports**.

9. You are aware that the antibiotics have been ordered for Harry George because of his leg infection. You decide to check the WBC results because you are curious (also, you are sure your nursing instructor will ask you about it). Document the WBC results for the times specified below and indicate whether each result is normal, elevated, or decreased.

Tests	Monday 1500	Tuesday 1100	Normal, Elevated, or Decreased?
Total WBC			
Neutrophil Segs			
Neutrophil Bands			
Lymphocytes			
Monocytes			
Eosinophils			
Basophils			

10. Assessing the data in the above table, explain what the results mean, including the direction of the change in the WBC and the significance of this change.

 • Click on **Return to Nurses' Station**.
   • Click on **Patient List**.
   • Click on **Get Report** for Harry George. Review the report.

11. Is there anything else you wish the nurse would have included in the report regarding osteomyelitis? If so, what?

 • Click on **Return to Nurses' Station**.
   • Click on **Medication Room**.
   • Click on **IV storage**.
   • Click on the **Small Volume** bin and choose the IV antibiotic that is due to be given at 0800.

12. What dilution of this IV antibiotic is available for you to administer?

13. Over what amount of time should you infuse the IV antibiotic? (*Hint:* For help, return to the Nurses' Station and click on the **Drug Guide** on the counter or click on the **Drug** icon in the lower left corner of your screen.)

14. If you are using an IV pump to deliver this medication piggyback, what rate (mL per hour) will you select to give this infusion?

Exercise 3

 CD-ROM Activity

 40 minutes

- Sign in to work at Pacific View Regional Hospital for Period of Care 2. (*Note:* If you are already in the virtual hospital from a previous exercise, click on **Leave the Floor** and then **Restart the Program** to get to the sign-in window.)
- From the Patient List, select Harry George (Room 401).
- Click on **Go to Nurses' Station** and then on **401** to enter Harry George's room.
- Inside the room, click on **Take Vital Signs**.

1. Record the vital sign findings below.

BP	SpO$_2$	Temp	HR	RR	Pain

- Click on **Patient Care**.
- Click on **Lower Extremities**.

2. Complete a focused neurovascular and skin assessment of the lower extremities and document your results below.

- Click on **Nurse-Client Interactions**.
- Select and view the video titled **1120: Wound Management**. (*Note:* If this video is not available, check the virtual clock to see whether enough time has elapsed. The video cannot be viewed before its specified time.)

3. How does the nurse describe the progress of Harry George's wound condition? How does the patient respond?

• Click on **Chart** and then on **401** for Harry George's record.
• Click on **Consultations**.

4. Describe the findings and impressions of the Wound Care Team Consult.

5. What was the recommended plan of care for the wound?

 6. Do you have any concerns regarding the above wound care? What different approach might you suggest? (*Hint:* See pages 409-410 in the textbook.)

7. What type of nutritional support would be appropriate to enhance wound healing?

 • Click on **Return to Room 401**.
• Click on **Medication Room**.
• Click on **MAR** to determine what medications you need to administer to Harry George during this time period (1115-1200).
• Click on **Return to Medication Room**.
• Click on **IV Storage**.

- Click on the **Small Volume** bin and choose the IV antibiotic that is due to be given at 1200.
- Prepare medication by clicking **Put Medication in Tray**.
- Click on **Close Bin**.
- Click on **View Medication Room**.
- Click on the **Drug** icon in the lower left corner of your screen.

8. Look up gentamicin in the Drug Guide. What must you first assess before administering this drug? (*Hint:* Look at alert under Administration and Handling.)

- Click on **Return to Medication Room**.
- Click on **Nurses' Station**.
- Click on **Chart** and then on **401** for Harry George's record.
- Click on **Laboratory Reports**.

9. What are Harry George's most recent peak and trough levels?

10. What should your nursing actions be based on these results?

11. For what toxic side effects must you monitor?

12. If Harry George's infection does not respond to the antibiotic therapy, or the wound does not heal, what adjunctive treatment would most likely be planned? (*Hint:* See page 414 in the textbook.) Explain how this would benefit Harry George.

LESSON 14

Malnutrition/Obesity

 Reading Assignment: Assessment of Nutrition and the Digestive System (Chapter 30)
Management of Clients with Malnutrition (Chapter 31)

Patients: Harry George, Room 401
Piya Jordan, Room 403
Jacqueline Catanazaro, Room 402

Goal: Utilize the nursing process to competently care for patients with nutritional disorders.

Objectives:

1. Identify patients at risk for malnutrition.
2. Perform a nutritional screening assessment on assigned patients.
3. Evaluate laboratory findings in relation to a patient's nutritional status.
4. Plan appropriate dietary interventions for a patient with malnutrition.
5. Identify a patient's risk factors related to obesity.
6. Formulate an appropriate patient education plan for an overweight patient.

In this lesson you will learn the essentials of caring for patients with nutritional disorders. You will explore each patient's history, perform a nutritional screening assessment, evaluate findings, and plan appropriate nursing interventions, including the patient's educational needs. Harry George is a 54-year-old male with a 4-year history of type 2 diabetes admitted with infection and swelling of his left foot. Piya Jordan is a 68-year-old female admitted with nausea and vomiting for several days following weeks of poor appetite and increasing weakness. Jacqueline Catanazaro is a 45-year-old female admitted with an acute exacerbation of asthma.

Exercise 1

 Clinical Preparation: Writing Activity

5 minutes

1. What are the average caloric and protein needs of a healthy adult?

2. What is the DRI? Identify its components.

Exercise 2

 CD-ROM Activity

 40 minutes

- Sign in to work at Pacific View Regional Hospital for Period of Care 1. (*Note:* If you are already in the virtual hospital from a previous exercise, click on **Leave the Floor** and then **Restart the Program** to get to the sign-in window.)
- From the Patient List, select Harry George (Room 401).
- Click on **Go to Nurses' Station**.
- Click on **Chart** and then on **401**.
- Click on **History and Physical**.

1. What risk factors for malnutrition are noted in Harry George's H&P?

- Click on **Return to Nurses' Station**.
- Click on **Chart** and then on **403** for Piya Jordan's record.
- Click on **History and Physical**.

2. What risk factors for malnutrition are noted in Piya Jordan's H&P?

- Click on **Return to Nurses' Station**.
- Click on **401** to enter Harry George's room.
- Click on **Patient Care**.

3. Although not every patient needs a complete nutritional assessment, it is essential to assess at-risk patients for symptoms of malnutrition. Referring to pages 671-682 of your textbook, assess Harry George for any of the identified findings associated with malnutrition. Obtain subjective information by reading the History and Physical, Nursing Admission, and Laboratory Reports in his chart. Obtain the objective data by completing a physical assessment in his room. Document your findings in column 2 below and on the next page. (*Note:* You will perform a similar assessment on Piya Jordan during Exercise 3 and record those findings in column 3.)

Screening Assessments	Harry George	Piya Jordan
Health History Biographic and demographic data		
Current Health Chief complaint related to nutrition		
Symptom analysis		
Past Health History Major illnesses and hospitalizations		
Medications and dietary supplements		
Allergies		
Family health history		
Psychosocial history		

Screening Assessments	Harry George	Piya Jordan

Physical Examination
Height and weight

Body mass index

Mouth

Abdomen

Laboratory Tests
Serum albumin

4. Evaluate the results of your findings in question 3. Is Harry George malnourished or at risk for malnutrition? Explain how you came to your conclusion.

5. What other anthropometric measures would be helpful in clarifying Harry George's nutritional status?

6. How will Harry George's nutritional status affect the healing of his left foot wound?

Exercise 3

 CD-ROM Activity

 40 minutes

- Sign in to work at Pacific View Regional Hospital for Period of Care 1. (*Note:* If you are already in the virtual hospital from a previous exercise, click on **Leave the Floor** and then **Restart the Program** to get to the sign-in window.)
- From the Patient List, select Harry George (Room 401) and Piya Jordan (Room 403).
- Click on **Go to Nurses' Station** and then on **403** to enter Piya Jordan's room.
- Click on **Patient Care**.

 1. Now perform the same nutritional screening assessment on Piya Jordan. Referring to pages 671-682 of your textbook, assess Piya Jordan for any of the identified findings associated with malnutrition. Obtain subjective information by reading the History and Physical, Nursing Admission, and Laboratory Reports in her chart. Obtain the objective data by completing a physical assessment in her room. Document your findings in column 3 of the table in Exercise 2, question 3.

 • Click on **Chart** and then on **403** for Piya Jordan's record.
- Click on **Physician's Orders**.

2. What is Piya Jordan's current GI status and diet?

3. Evaluate the results of your findings from questions 1 and 2. Is Piya Jordan malnourished or at risk for malnutrition? Explain how you came to your conclusion.

4. Compare and contrast your findings for Harry George and Piya Jordan. What are the similarities? What are the differences?

5. What other laboratory tests would give you more information on the nutritional status of these two patients?

6. Identify two nursing diagnosis related to Piya Jordan's and Harry George's malnourished status.

7. Read the Evidence-Based Practice in Action box on page 692 of your textbook. How do these findings relate to Piya Jordan?

Exercise 4

 CD-ROM Activity

 30 minutes

- Sign in to work at Pacific View Regional Hospital for Period of Care 2. (*Note:* If you are already in the virtual hospital from a previous exercise, click on **Leave the Floor** and then **Restart the Program** to get to the sign-in window.)
- From the Patient List, select Jacqueline Catanazaro (Room 402).
- Click on **Go to Nurses' Station**.
- Click on **Chart** and then on **402** for Jacqueline Catanazaro's record.
- Click on **Nursing Admission**.

1. Document Jacqueline Catanazaro's current height and weight below.

2. Calculate Jacqueline Catanazaro's BMI. (*Hint:* See page 677 in your textbook for the formula.)

3. Is Jacqueline Catanazaro's nutritional status normal, overweight, obese, or morbidly obese? (*Hint:* See page 677 in the textbook.)

→ • Click on **History and Physical**.

4. What complication of obesity does Jacqueline Catanazaro suffer from?

5. What other complications is she at risk for?

6. What are the contributing factors for Jacqueline Catanazaro's increased weight?

→ • Click on **Return to Nurses' Station**.
  • Click on **MAR** and then on tab **402** for Jacqueline Catanazaro's record.

7. Do any of the medications ordered for Jacqueline Catanazaro cause weight gain? If so, explain. (*Hint:* For help, return to the Nurses' Station and click on the **Drug Guide** on the counter or click on the **Drug** icon in the lower left corner of your screen.)

• Click on **Return to Nurses' Station** and then on **402** to enter the patient's room.
  • Inside the room, click on **Patient Care** and then on **Nurse-Client Interactions**.
  • Select and view the video titled **1140: Compliance—Medications**. (*Note:* If this video is not available, check the virtual clock to see whether enough time has elapsed. The video cannot be viewed before its specified time.)

8. What concern does Jacqueline Catanazaro voice regarding her medications?

9. Evaluate the nurse's response. Was it appropriate? Accurate?

10. What else could the nurse have suggested to help Jacqueline Catanazaro lose weight?

11. If Jacqueline Catanazaro had been severely obese (BMI greater than 40), what other treatment options might she have? Briefly explain these options.

LESSON **15**

Intestinal Obstruction/ Colorectal Cancer

Reading Assignment: Management of Clients with Intestinal Disorders (Chapter 35)

Patient: Piya Jordan, Room 403

Goal: Utilize the nursing process to competently care for patients with intestinal disorders.

Objectives:

1. Correlate a patient's history and clinical manifestations with a diagnosis of intestinal obstruction.
2. Evaluate laboratory and diagnostic test results of a patient admitted with an intestinal disorder.
3. Plan appropriate nursing interventions for a patient with a nasogastric tube.
4. Prioritize nursing care for a patient with an intestinal obstruction.
5. Provide appropriate psychosocial interventions for a patient and family diagnosed with colon cancer.
6. Formulate an appropriate patient education plan for a postoperative patient with colorectal cancer.

In this lesson you will learn the essentials of caring for a patient admitted with an intestinal obstruction and diagnosed with colorectal cancer. You will explore the patient's history, evaluate presenting symptoms and treatment, plan appropriate nursing interventions, and develop an individualized teaching plan. Piya Jordan is a 68-year-old female admitted with nausea and vomiting for several days following weeks of poor appetite and increasing weakness.

Exercise 1

 Clinical Preparation: Writing Activity

20 minutes

1. Describe the pathophysiology of fluid and electrolyte imbalances associated with an intestinal obstruction.

2. Identify and briefly describe the three categories of etiology related to intestinal obstruction.

3. How does the removal of polyps help to prevent colorectal cancer?

4. Identify the most likely sites of bloodborne metastasis for colorectal cancer.

Exercise 2

 CD-ROM Activity

 40 minutes

- Sign in to work at Pacific View Regional Hospital for Period of Care 1. (*Note:* If you are already in the virtual hospital from a previous exercise, click on **Leave the Floor** and then **Restart the Program** to get to the sign-in window.)
- From the Patient List, select Piya Jordan (Room 403).
- Click on **Go to Nurses' Station**.
- Click on **Chart** and then on **403**.
- Click on **Emergency Department**.

1. What were Piya Jordan's presenting symptoms?

 - Click on **History and Physical**.

2. What history of symptoms is recorded?

 - Click on **Laboratory Reports**.

3. Document Piya Jordan's admission electrolyte results below. Evaluate whether each result is normal, decreased, or increased. Provide rationales for any abnormalities in the last column.

	Monday 2200	Decreased, Normal, or Increased?	Rationale for Abnormality
Sodium			
Potassium			
Chloride			
CO_2			
Creatinine			
BUN			
Amylase			

→ • Click on **Diagnostic Reports**.

4. What was the result of the KUB? What do Piya Jordan's air-fluid levels (gas shadows) indicate?

5. Why was a CT scan of the abdomen ordered? What was the result?

6. What part of the bowel is the terminal ileum?

7. Was Piya Jordan's obstruction mechanical, neurogenic, or vascular? Explain.

8. If Piya Jordan had sought medical attention before the obstruction worsened, what other diagnostic testing might she have undergone? Explain what the test would show.

→ • Click on **History and Physical**.

9. Now that you know Piya Jordan has a colonic mass, let's look at those presenting symptoms again. Common clinical manifestations of colorectal cancer are listed below. Place an X next to each sign or symptom consistent with Piya Jordan's history and her physical examination findings on admission.

    _____ a. Rectal bleeding   _____ i. Ribbonlike stools

    _____ b. Changed bowel habits   _____ j. Abdominal pain and cramping

    _____ c. Blood in stools   _____ k. Palpable mass

    _____ d. Anemia   _____ l. Abdominal distention

    _____ e. Straining to pass stools _____ m. Weight loss

    _____ f. Anorexia   _____ n. Weakness

    _____ g. Nausea and vomiting   _____ o. Debility

    _____ h. Fatigue

→ • Click on **Physician's Orders**.

10. What IV fluid did the ED physician initially order? Why? (*Hint:* Look at vital signs in Emergency Department Record and relate to fluid/electrolyte changes noted with intestinal obstruction.)

11. What else did the ED physician order to treat the intestinal obstruction? Explain the purpose of this intervention.

 • Click on **Return to Nurses' Station**.
• Click on **403** to enter Piya Jordan's room.
• Click on **Patient Care**.

12. Perform a focused abdominal assessment. Document your findings below.

13. Describe any additional assessments and/or interventions related to the NGT that you might do for Piya Jordan.

Exercise 3

 CD-ROM Activity

 45 minutes

- Sign in to work at Pacific View Regional Hospital for Period of Care 3. (*Note:* If you are already in the virtual hospital from a previous exercise, click on **Leave the Floor** and then **Restart the Program** to get to the sign-in window.)
- From the Patient List, select Piya Jordan (Room 403).
- Click on **Go to Nurses' Station**.
- Click on **Chart** and then on **403** for Piya Jordan's chart.
- Click on **History and Physical**.

1. Below is a list of risk factors for colorectal cancer. Place an X next to any that are documented in Piya Jordan's record.

_____ a. Age

_____ b. History of polyps

_____ c. High-fat, low-residue diet

_____ d. Inflammatory bowel disease

_____ e. Family history

_____ f. History of breast, ovarian, or endometrial cancer

→ • Click on **Laboratory Reports**.

2. Below, document Piya Jordan's admission H&H. How would you explain the results?

	Monday 2200	Decreased, WNL, or Increased?	Rationale for Abnormality
Hemoglobin			
Hematocrit			

→ • Click on **Expired MARs**.

3. What was administered preoperatively to clean out Piya Jordan's bowel?

4. If Piya Jordan's surgery had not been an emergency, what type of bowel prep would you have expected to administer? Why is this done?

→ • Click on **Surgical Reports**.

5. Review the operative report. Name and describe the surgical procedure.

6. If the tumor had been larger, what further surgery might Piya Jordan have needed? (*Hint:* See Table 60-2 in your textbook.)

7. What is the most likely cell type for Piya Jordan's cancer?

8. How will the physician know what kind of cancer the tumor is?

9. How would you classify Piya Jordan's tumor according to the Dukes' classification system? Explain.

→ • Click on **Laboratory Results**.

10. Why did the physician order an amylase, lipase, and LFTs? What do the results demonstrate?

→ • Click on **Return to Nurses' Station**.
   • Click on **403** to enter Piya Jordan's room.
   • Click on **Patient Care**.
   • Click on **Nurse-Client Interactions**.
   • Select and view the video titled **1500: Preventing Complications**. (*Note:* If this video is not available, check the virtual clock to see whether enough time has elapsed. The video cannot be viewed before its specified time.)

11. What nursing interventions are discussed during this brief video? Why are they appropriate for Piya Jordan?

→ • Now select and view the video titled **1500: Discharge Planning**.

12. The daughter seems to be overwhelmed by her mother's illness and needs. Describe psychosocial interventions that the nurse might plan to help Piya Jordan and her daughter.

13. What would you teach the daughter regarding health promotion and preventing colon cancer in herself?

14. Identify teaching points that should be discussed with Piya Jordan before her discharge.

LESSON **16** ────────────────────────

Diabetes Mellitus, Part 1

──────────────────────────────────

Reading Assignment: Management of Clients with Diabetes Mellitus (Chapter 47)

Patient: Harry George, Room 401

Goal: Utilize the nursing process to competently care for patients with diabetes mellitus.

Objectives:

1. Describe the pathophysiology of diabetes mellitus.
2. Compare and contrast the characteristics of type 1 and type 2 diabetes.
3. Identify the relationship between diabetes and other disease processes.
4. Evaluate a patient's risk factors for diabetes.
5. Assess a patient for short- and long-term complications of diabetes.
6. Develop an appropriate plan of care for a patient with type 2 diabetes.

In this lesson you will learn the essentials of caring for a patient admitted with complications related to diabetes mellitus. You will explore the patient's history, evaluate presenting symptoms and treatment, plan appropriate nursing interventions, and develop an individualized teaching plan. Harry George is a 54-year-old male with a 4-year history of type 2 diabetes admitted with infection and swelling of his left foot.

Exercise 1

Clinical Preparation: Writing Activity

20 minutes

1. Describe the pathophysiology of diabetes mellitus and the basis for the resulting abnormalities in carbohydrate, protein, and fat utilization.

2. Briefly define and summarize the etiologic differences between type 1 and type 2 diabetes mellitus.

3. Compare and contrast the distinquishing features of type 1 and type 2 diabetes mellitus (DM) by completing the chart below.

Features	Type 1 DM	Type 2 DM
Synonyms		
Age at onset		
Incidence		
Types of onset		
Endogenous insulin production		
Body weight at onset		
HLA antigens		
Antibodies		
Manifestations		
Treatment		

Exercise 2

 CD-ROM Activity

 35 minutes

- Sign in to work at Pacific View Regional Hospital for Period of Care 1. (*Note:* If you are already in the virtual hospital from a previous exercise, click on **Leave the Floor** and then **Restart the Program** to get to the sign-in window.)
- From the Patient List, select Harry George (Room 401).
- Click on **Go to Nurses' Station**.
- Click on **Chart** and then on **401** for Harry George's record.
- Click on **History and Physical**.

1. What risk factors for diabetes are noted in Harry George's history?

2. Describe the history of this patient's present illness.

3. What is the relationship between the infection in Harry George's foot and his diabetes mellitus? (*Hint:* Read about chronic complications in the textbook.)

- Click on **Laboratory Reports**.

4. What was Harry George's admitting blood glucose level?

5. What abnormalities in Harry George's urinalysis results can be attributed to diabetes? Explain the relationship.

→ • Click on **Emergency Department**.

6. What factor in Harry George's recent history most likely contributed to his hyperglycemia? (*Hint:* Read ED physician's notes for 1345.)

7. Listed below are clinical manifestations of diabetes mellitus identified in the textbook. In column 2, indicate (with Yes or No) whether each manifestation is usually present in type 2 diabetes. Then indicate (with Yes or No) whether Harry George displays each manifestation based on the nurse's initial assessment.

Clinical Manifestations	Present in Type 2 DM? (Yes or No)	Experienced by Harry George? (Yes or No)
Polyuria		
Polydispia		
Polyphagia		
Recurrent blurred vision		
Weakness, fatigue, dizziness		
Weight Loss		
Ketonuria		
Pruritus, skin infections		

8. To what extent does Harry George fit the typical picture of a patient with type 2 diabetes mellitus?

 • Click on **Return to Nurses' Station**.
   • Click on **401** to enter Harry George's room.
   • Click on **Patient Care**.
   • Click on **Nurse-Client Interactions**.
   • Select and view the video titled **0755: Disease Management**. (*Note:* If this video is not available, check the virtual clock to see whether enough time has elapsed. The video cannot be viewed before its specified time.)

9. What does Harry George tell the nurse about his appetite?

 • Click on **Chart** and then on **401**.
   • Click on **Physician's Orders**.

10. What diet has been ordered for the patient?

 11. Describe the current recommended nutritional guidelines for the patient with diabetes mellitus. (*Hint:* See Table 47-4 in your textbook.)

12. How might the patient's alcohol intake affect his blood glucose levels?

Exercise 3

 CD-ROM Activity

 40 minutes

- Sign in to work at Pacific View Regional Hospital for Period of Care 2. (*Note:* If you are already in the virtual hospital from a previous exercise, click on **Leave the Floor** and then **Restart the Program** to get to the sign-in window.)
- From the Patient List, select Harry George (Room 401).
- Click on **Go to Nurses' Station**.
- Click on **Chart** and then on **401** for Harry George's record.
- Click on **Physician's Orders**.

1. What test is ordered that can be used to determine Harry George's control of diabetes mellitus? Describe the purpose of this test. How often should it be done?

2. What was the result of this test for Harry George? Evaluate and explain how well controlled his diabetes is based on these results.

3. What implication does the patient's issue of poor glycemic control have for his future?

4. How could Harry George's alcohol intake affect his $HgbA_{1c}$ test result? What implications does this have in managing Harry George's diabetes? How should the nurse intervene?

• Click on **Return to Nurses' Station**.
- Click on **401** to enter Harry George's room.
- Click on **Patient Care**.

5. Perform a head-to-toe assessment on Harry George. Document any abnormal results below.

Assessment Area	Assessment Results
Head & Neck	
Chest	
Back & Spine	
Upper Extremities	
Abdomen	
Pelvic	
Lower Extremities	

 • Click on **EPR** and then on **Login**.
- In the upper left corner of your screen, select **401** as the patient's room and **Neurologic** as the category.

6. List any abnormal information obtained from the neurologic data recorded on Monday at 1835.

7. Describe the following potential long-term complications for diabetes mellitus.

Coronary artery disease

Cerebrovascular disease

Hypertension

Peripheral vascular disease

Retinopathy

Nephropathy

Neuropathy

8. Does Harry George exhibit any signs or symptoms that would alert you to the possibility of any of the long-term complications noted in question 6? If so, explain. (*Hint:* Review your responses to questions 4 and 5 and consider your response to question 5 in Exercise 2.)

9. What patient teaching would you plan to offer Harry George to prevent injury secondary to reduced sensation in his left foot? (*Hint:* See Chart 68-8 in your textbook.)

LESSON 17

Diabetes Mellitus, Part 2

 Reading Assignment: Management of Clients with Diabetes Mellitus (Chapter 47)

Patient: Harry George, Room 401

Goal: Utilize the nursing process to competently administer medications prescribed to treat patients with diabetes mellitus.

Objectives:

1. Describe the pharmacologic therapy used for a patient with diabetes.
2. Evaluate a patient's response to insulin therapy.
3. Assess a patient for side effects of insulin therapy.
4. Describe the clinical manifestations of hypoglycemia as a side effect of insulin therapy.
5. Develop an individualized teaching plan for a patient with type 2 diabetes.

In this lesson you will learn the essentials regarding pharmacologic therapy for a patient admitted with complications related to diabetes mellitus. You will identify, describe, administer, and evaluate effects of prescribed antidiabetic medications. Harry George is a 54-year-old male with a 4-year history of type 2 diabetes admitted with infection and swelling of his left foot.

Exercise 1

Clinical Preparation: Writing Activity

30 minutes

1. Identify and describe the various types of insulin by completing the table below and on the next page.

Insulin Classification/ Generic Name	Brand Name(s)	Onset	Peak	Duration
Rapid-Acting/ Aspart				
Lispro				

Insulin Classification/ Generic Name	Brand Name(s)	Onset	Peak	Duration
Short-Acting/ Regular insulin				
Intermediate-Acting/ NPH				
Lente				
Long-Acting/ Ultralente				
Glargine				

2. Below, identify the five classifications of oral hypoglycemic agents and describe the mechanism of action for each. (*Hint:* See Integrating Pharmacology Box on page 1254 of your textbook.)

Classification	Mechanism of Action
a.	
b.	
c.	
d.	
e.	

Exercise 2

 CD-ROM Activity

 40 minutes

- Sign in to work at Pacific View Regional Hospital for Period of Care 1. (*Note:* If you are already in the virtual hospital from a previous exercise, click on **Leave the Floor** and then **Restart the Program** to get to the sign-in window.)
- From the Patient List, select Harry George (Room 401).
- Click on **Go to Nurses' Station**.
- Click on **Chart** and then on **401** for Harry George's record.
- Click on **Emergency Department**.

1. What medication was ordered to control Harry George's diabetes?

2. How would you give the IV insulin? (*Hint:* For help, return to the Nurses' Station and click on the **Drug** icon in the lower left corner of the screen.)

3. Look at ED physician progress notes for Monday at 1345. What does the physician plan to order for the sliding scale insulin coverage?

 • Click on **Physician's Orders**.

4. Look at the orders for the same time frame. What was the actual sliding scale insulin order?

→ • Click on **Return to Nurses' Station**.
  • Click on **Kardex** and then on tab **401** for Harry George's record.

5. According to the Kardex, how often should the capillary blood glucose be tested?

→ • Click on **Return to Nurses' Station**.
  • Click on **MAR** and then on tab **401** for Harry George's record.

6. According to the MAR, when should the insulin sliding scale should be administered? What was the time of this order?

7. What would you do regarding the inconsistencies identified above?

8. What problems might you anticipate for Harry George if he does not receive insulin coverage at bedtime?

→ • Click on **Return to Nurses' Station**.
  • Click on **401** to enter Harry George's room.
  • Click on **Clinical Alerts**.

9. What is the clinical alert for 0730?

Prepare and administer the sliding scale insulin for this glucose level by following these steps:

- Click **Medication Room** on the bottom of the screen.
- Click **MAR** or **Review MAR** at any time to verify how much insulin to administer based on sliding scale. (*Hint:* Remember to look at the patient name on the MAR to make sure you have the correct patient's records—you must click on correct room number within the MAR.) Click on **Return to Medication Room** after reviewing the correct MAR.
- Click on **Unit Dosage** and then on drawer **401** for Harry George's medications.
- Select **Insulin Regular**; next, click on **Put Medication on Tray** and then on **Close Drawer**.
- Click **View Medication Room**.
- Click on **Preparation** and choose the correct medication to administer. Click **Prepare**.
- Click **Next**, choose the correct patient to administer this medication to, and click **Finish**.
- You can click on **Review Your Medications** and then on **Return to Medication Room** when ready. Once you are back in the Medication Room, you may go directly to Harry George's room by clicking on **401** at the bottom of the screen.
- Click on **Patient Care**.
- Click on **Medication Administration** and follow the steps in the Administration Wizard to complete the insulin administration.

10. How much insulin should be administered?

11. What is the preferred site of administration for fastest absorption?

12. Fill in the table below regarding the insulin you just administered.

	Expected Length of Time	Actual Time After 0730 Dose
Onset		
Peak		
Duration		

13. At what time would Harry George be at most risk for hypoglycemia? Describe the clinical manifestations that would indicate this acute complication.

14. While you are preparing to administer Harry George's insulin, he asks you why he is taking this since he did not use insulin at home. How would you answer him?

15. For what side effects should you monitor Harry George related to his insulin regimen? (*Hint:* For help, click on the **Drug** icon in the lower left corner of the Nurses' Station screen.)

Exercise 3

 CD-ROM Activity

 40 minutes

• Sign in to work at Pacific View Regional Hospital for Period of Care 4. (*Note:* If you are already in the virtual hospital from a previous exercise, click on **Leave the Floor** and then **Restart the Program** to get to the sign-in window.)
• From the Patient List, select Harry George (Room 401).
• Click on **Go to Nurses' Station**.
• Click on **Chart** and then on **401** for Harry George's record.
• Click on **Nurse's Notes**.

1. Read the notes for Wednesday at 1730. What does the patient request regarding glyburide?

2. How would you respond to the patient's demands?

3. How often did Harry George take the glyburide at home?

4. Why do you think this was increased in the hospital? What concerns might you have regarding this increase? (*Hint:* Patient is also receiving insulin.)

5. What classification of oral hypoglycemics does glyburide belong to? (*Hint:* For help, return to the Nurses' Station and click on the **Drug Guide** on the counter or on the **Drug** icon in the lower left corner of your screen.)

6. For what side effects of glyburide should you assess Harry George? (*Hint:* Consult the Drug Guide.)

7. What specific patient teaching points should you give Harry George regarding glyburide?

➡ • Click on **Go to Nurses' Station**.
   • Click on **Chart** and then on **401** for Harry George's record.
   • Click on **Laboratory Reports**.

8. Below, chart Harry George's blood glucose levels and insulin administration since admission to the medical-surgical unit. (*Hint:* You may have to review the expired MARs in the chart to verify whether insulin was given for HS glucose measurement on Tuesday.)

Date/Time	Blood Glucose Level	Amount of Regular Insulin Administered

9. Considering Harry George's pattern of blood glucose levels, would you evaluate his current therapy as effective? If not, how might the physician further treat this patient's diabetes?

10. If you were reviewing the chart on Wednesday evening and found the information recorded in the table in question 8, what concern would you ethically and legally be bound to report?

LESSON **18** ─────────────────────────

Hypertension

───────────────────────────────────────

⟋⟋⟋ **Reading Assignment:** Management of Clients with Hypertensive Disorders
(Chapter 54)

Patients: Patricia Newman, Room 406
Harry George, Room 401

Goal: Utilize the nursing process to competently care for patients with hypertension.

Objectives:

1. Describe the four classifications of blood pressure.
2. Identify the presence of risk factors for hypertension in assigned patients.
3. Discuss pharmacologic therapies available to treat hypertension.
4. Perform appropriate assessments prior to administering pharmacologic therapy for hypertension.
5. Develop an extensive educational plan for patients with hypertension.

In this lesson you will learn the essentials of caring for a patient with hypertension. You will explore the patient's history, evaluate presenting symptoms and treatment, identify blood pressure classification, provide appropriate nursing interventions, and plan an appropriate patient education plan related to the hypertension. Patricia Newman is a 61-year-old female admitted with pneumonia and a history of emphysema. Harry George is a 54-year-old male admitted with infection and swelling of the left foot.

Exercise 1

 Clinical Preparation: Writing Activity

 20 minutes

1. Identify and describe the four classifications of blood pressure.

2. Describe the pathophysiologic factors that contribute to the development of hypertension.

3. Define the following terms.

   a. Primary hypertension

b. Secondary hypertension

c. White coat hypertension

d. Isolated systolic hypertension (ISH)

e. Persistent severe hypertension or resistant hypertension (formerly called *malignant hypertension*)

4. Identify four nonmodifiable risk factors for hypertension.

5. Identify six modifiable risk factors for hypertension.

Exercise 2

 CD-ROM Activity

 45 minutes

- Sign in to work at Pacific View Regional Hospital for Period of Care 1. (*Note:* If you are already in the virtual hospital from a previous exercise, click on **Leave the Floor** and then **Restart the Program** to get to the sign-in window.)
- From the Patient List, select Patricia Newman (Room 406).
- Click on **Go to Nurses' Station**.
- Click on **Chart** and then on **406** for Patricia Newman's chart.
- Click on **History and Physical**.

1. How long has Patricia Newman been diagnosed with hypertension?

 • Click on **Nursing Admission**.

2. What risk factors for hypertension does Patricia Newman have?

 • Click on **Physician's Orders**.

3. In the table below, identify the two medications ordered to treat Patricia Newman's hypertension. For each one, identify the drug classification and mechanism of action. You will complete the table in questions 4 and 5. (*Hint:* You may consult the Drug Guide in the Nurses' Station.)

Medication	Drug Classification	Mechanism of Action	Nursing Assessments	Common Side Effects

➤ • Click on **Return to Nurses' Station**.
  • Click on the **Drug Guide** on the desk.

4. What nursing assessments are important before administering the medications you identified in question 3? Record your answer in the fourth column of the table.

5. For what side effects will the nurse need to monitor the patient? Record you answer in the last column of the table.

➤ • Click on **Return to Nurses' Station**; then select **EPR** and click on **Login**. Choose **406** from the Patient drop-down menu. Review the vital sign findings.

6. What are Patricia Newman's documented blood pressure measurements since admission?

7. Is her prescribed antihypertensive medication currently effective?

8. In what classification would you put Patricia Newman's blood pressure based on her most current readings? Explain.

➤ • Click on **Exit EPR**.
  • Click on **406** to go to Patricia Newman's room.
  • Click on **Patient Care**.
  • Click on **Nurse-Client Interactions**.
  • Select and view the video titled **0740: Evaluation: Response to Care**. (*Note:* If this video is not available, check the virtual clock to see whether enough time has elapsed. The video cannot be viewed before its specified time.)

9. What might be contributing to Patricia Newman's currently elevated blood pressure?

➤ • Click on **Chart** and then on **406** for Patricia Newman's record.
  • Click on **History and Physical**.

10. What indicates that Patricia Newman is in need of further teaching regarding hypertension?

→ • Click on **Patient Education**.

11. What additional educational goals would be appropriate for Patricia Newman?

12. Develop a comprehensive individualized teaching plan for Patricia Newman regarding nonpharmacologic measures to treat hypertension.

• Click on **Nursing Admission**.

13. Was Patricia Newman following any of the interventions you identified in question 12 to reduce her blood pressure at home? Explain.

 • Click on **Physician's Orders**.

14. Identify any of the interventions addressed in question 12 that were ordered for Patricia Newman during this hospital stay.

15. As the nurse caring for Patricia Newman, what do you think would be your professional responsibility related to your findings for questions 13 and 14?

Exercise 3

 CD-ROM Activity

 40 minutes

- Sign in to work at Pacific View Regional Hospital for Period of Care 1. (*Note:* If you are already in the virtual hospital from a previous exercise, click on **Leave the Floor** and then **Restart the Program** to get to the sign-in window.)
- From the Patient List, select Harry George (Room 401).
- Click on **Go to Nurses' Station**.
- Click on **EPR** and then on **Login**.
- Select **401** for the patient's room and **Vital Signs** as the category.

1. Document Harry George's blood pressures (BP) below.

	Tues 0305	Tues 0705	Tues 1105	Tues 1505	Tues 1905	Tues 2305	Wed 0305	Wed 0705
BP								

→ • Click on **Exit EPR**.
  • Click on **Chart** and then on **401** for Harry George's records.
  • Click on **History and Physical**.

2. Does Harry George have a history of hypertension?

3. Does he have any risk factors for hypertension? If yes, please identify.

4. Based on the BP recordings in question 1, in what classification would you put Harry George's blood pressure?

5. For what potential target organ damage should you assess related to untreated hypertension?

→ • Click on **Return to Nurses' Station**.
  • Click on **401**.
  • Click on **Patient Care**.
  • Select the various assessment areas (yellow buttons) and system subcategories (green buttons) as needed to answer question 6.

6. Listed below are physical assessment findings indicative of target organ damage from hypertension. Place an X next to any of the following findings that you noted during your physical assessment of Harry George.

_____   a. Distended neck veins

_____   b. Enlarged thyroid

_____   c. Dysrhythmias

_____   d. Murmurs

_____   e. Abdominal bruit

_____   f. Edema

_____   g. Carotid bruits

_____   h. Increased heart rate

_____   i. Precordial impulses

_____   j. S_3 and S_4 heart sounds

_____   k. Diminished or absent peripheral pulses

_____   l. Bilateral inequality of pulses

7. What target organ disease is consistent with the above findings?

8. Several diagnostic tests were ordered by the physician. Although these tests may have been ordered for various purposes, they may specifically help to identify target organ disease. In the middle column below, indicate how each test might be helpful. (*Note:* You will complete this table in questions 7 and 8.)

Diagnostic Test	How Test Might Help Identify Target Organ Disease	Results
Chest x-ray		
BUN		
Creatinine		
Urinalysis		

→ • Click on **Diagnostic Reports**.

9. Record the results of Harry George's chest x-ray in the third column of the table in question 8 and indicate whether the results suggest the presence of target organ disease.

→ • Click on **Laboratory Reports**.

10. Find and record the lab results for BUN, creatinine, and urinalysis in the table in question 8. Indicate what these results mean related to target organ disease.

11. What would be the first step in treating Harry George's hypertension?

12. If the above interventions failed to lower Harry George's blood pressure to normal limits, what classification of drugs might the health care provider prescribe?

13. If Harry George continues to have inadequate blood pressure control, describe the next two steps in hypertension management that may be used for this patient.

Atrial Fibrillation

/○ひ **Reading Assignment:** Assessment of the Cardiac System (Chapter 56)
Management of Clients with Dysrhythmias (Chapter 59)

Patients: Piya Jordan, Room 403

Goal: Utilize the nursing process to competently care for patients with dysrhythmias.

Objectives:

1. Describe telemetry rhythm strip characteristics of atrial fibrillation.
2. Identify potential etiologic causes of atrial fibrillation for assigned patient.
3. Assess patient for clinical manifestations of atrial fibrillation.
4. Develop plan of care to monitor patient for potential complications of atrial fibrillation
5. Perform appropriate assessments prior to administering pharmacologic therapy for atrial fibrillation.
6. Accurately administer IV digoxin.
7. Discuss the use of anticoagulation therapy for a patient with atrial fibrillation.
8. Develop appropriate educational outcome for a patient with a history of atrial fibrillation.

In this lesson you will learn the essentials of caring for a patient with a cardiac dysrhythmia. You will explore the patient's history, evaluate presenting symptoms and treatment, provide appropriate nursing interventions, and plan an appropriate patient educational outcome related to the dysrhythmia. Piya Jordan is a 68-year-old female admitted with nausea, vomiting, and abdominal pain.

Exercise 1

 Clinical Preparation: Writing Activity

 20 minutes

1. Briefly describe the three pathophysiologic mechanisms that can cause dysrhythmias.

   a.

   b.

   c.

2. Describe the concept of atrial kick. Why is this important?

3. Identify the cardiac event represented by each of the following waves and measured intervals.

   a. P wave

   b. QRS wave

c. T wave

d. PR interval

e. ST segment

f. QT interval

g. U wave

4. Describe the seven steps of ECG analysis.

a.

b.

c.

d.

e.

f.

g.

Exercise 2

 CD-ROM Activity

 35 minutes

- Sign in to work at Pacific View Regional Hospital for Period of Care 1. (*Note:* If you are already in the virtual hospital from a previous exercise, click on **Leave the Floor** and then **Restart the Program** to get to the sign-in window.)
- From the Patient List, select Piya Jordan (Room 403).
- Click on **Go to Nurses' Station**.
- Click on **403** to enter Piya Jordan's room.

1. What information regarding Piya Jordan's cardiovascular status is obtained on initial observation of patient?

2. What is telemetry monitoring?

3. What is atrial fibrillation?

4. Describe the rhythm strip you would expect to see on Piya Jordan's monitor.

5. How does this differ from normal sinus rhythm?

6. What effect does this rhythm have on cardiac output? Explain.

7. For what clinical manifestations related to atrial fibrillation should you monitor Piya Jordan?

→ • Click on **Patient Care** and perform a general assessment of Piya Jordan.

8. Are any of the symptoms you listed in question 7 present in Piya Jordan? If not, how would you explain that?

9. If Piya Jordan's heart rate increases, how might the atrial fibrillation affect her blood pressure? Describe the underlying physiology. (*Hint:* Think about the atrial kick.)

→ • Click on **Chart** and then on **403**.
• Click on **Diagnostic Reports**.

10. Did Piya Jordan have a 12-lead ECG done? If yes, what was the rhythm? If not, do you think it should have been done? Why or why not?

11. For what potential complications should you monitor Piya Jordan?

Exercise 3

 CD-ROM Activity

 45 minutes

• Sign in to work at Pacific View Regional Hospital for Period of Care 1. (*Note:* If you are already in the virtual hospital from a previous exercise, click on **Leave the Floor** and then **Restart the Program** to get to the sign-in window.)
• From the Patient List, select Piya Jordan (Room 403).
• Click on **Go to Nurses' Station**.
• Click on **MAR** and then on tab **403** for Piya Jordan's record.

1. What medication is prescribed to treat Piya Jordan's atrial fibrillation? Describe the pharmacodynamics of this medication as related to atrial fibrillation. (*Hint:* For help, return to the Nurses' Station and click on the **Drug Guide** on the counter or on the **Drug** icon in the lower left corner of your screen.)

2. Why did the physician order a digoxin level when the patient first presented to the ED? (*Hint:* Review her presenting symptoms, as well as the Drug Guide.)

→ • Click on **Return to Nurses' Station**.
   • Click on **Chart** and then on **403**.
   • Click on **Laboratory Reports**.

3. What was the digoxin level? Is this level therapeutic or toxic?

4. For what other symptoms would you monitor Piya Jordan in relation to digoxin toxicity?

→ • Click on **History and Physical**.

5. What other medication was Piya Jordan prescribed related to atrial fibrillation before this admission? Provide a rationale for this medication. (*Hint:* Think of potential serious complications of atrial fibrillation.)

→ • Click on **Physician's Orders**.

6. What two items did the physician prescribe preoperatively to reverse Piya Jordan's anti-coagulation? How would you know this was effective? Please explain.

7. What was ordered postoperatively to prevent clot formation?

→ • Click on **Nursing Admission**.

8. What knowledge (or lack of knowledge) does Piya Jordan verbalize regarding her history of atrial fibrillation? (*Hint:* Check the Health Promotion section.)

→ • Click on **Patient Education**.

9. What might you add to these outcomes relative to your answer to question 8?

10. What other treatment options are available to treat Piya Jordan's atrial fibrillation?

11. What interventional therapy may be used for patients with recurrent or sustained atrial fibrillation?

Medication Preparation

- Click on **Return to Nurses' Station**.
- Click on **Medication Room**.
- Click on **MAR** to determine medications that Piya Jordan is ordered to receive at 0800. (*Note:* You may click on **Review MAR** at any time to verify correct medication order. Remember to look at the patient name on the MAR to make sure you have the correct patient's record—you must click on the correct room number within the MAR. Click on **Return to Medication Room** after reviewing the correct MAR.)
- Based on your care for Piya Jordan, access the various storage areas of the Medication Room to obtain the necessary medications you need to administer.
- For each area you access, first select the medication you plan to administer, then click **Put Medication on Tray**. When finished with a storage area, click on **Close Drawer**.
- Click **View Medication Room**.
- Click on **Preparation** and choose the correct medication to administer. Click **Prepare**.
- Click **Next** and choose the correct patient to administer this medication to. Click **Finish**.
- Repeat the above two steps until all medications that you want to administer are prepared.
- You can click **Review Your Medications** and then **Return to Medication Room** when you are ready. Once you are back in the Medication Room, you may go directly to Piya Jordan's room by clicking on **403** at the bottom of the screen.

Medication Administration

- Administer the medication, utilizing the five rights of medication administration. After you have collected the appropriate assessment data and are ready for administration, click **Patient Care** and then **Medication Administration**. Verify that the correct patient and medication(s) appear in the left-hand window. Then click the down arrow next to Select. From the drop-down menu, select **Administer** and complete the Administration Wizard by providing any information requested. When the Wizard stops asking for information, click **Administer to Patient**. Specify **Yes** when asked whether this administration should be recorded in the MAR. Finally, click **Finish**.

12. Over how many minutes would you administer the IV digoxin?

13. What should you have assessed before administering digoxin to Piya Jordan today?

Now let's see how you did!

 • Click on **Leave the Floor** at the bottom of your screen. From the Floor Menu, select **Look at Your Preceptor's Evaluation**. Then click on **Medication Scorecard**.

14. Note below whether or not you correctly administered the appropriate medications. If not, why do you think you were incorrect? According to Table C in this scorecard, what resources should be used and what assessments should be completed before administering the medications? Did you use these resources and perform these assessments correctly?

LESSON **20** —————————————————————

Asthma

—————————————————————

👓 **Reading Assignment:** Management of Clients with Lower Airway and
Pulmonary Vessel Disorders (Chapter 63)

Patient: Jacqueline Catanazaro, Room 402

Goal: Utilize the nursing process to competently care for patients with asthma.

Objectives:

1. Identify clinical manifestations of an acute asthmatic exacerbation.
2. Evaluate diagnostic tests as they relate to a patient's oxygenation status.
3. Describe medications used to treat asthma, including mechanism of action and therapeutic effects.
4. Prioritize nursing care for a patient with an acute exacerbation of asthma.
5. Formulate an appropriate patient education plan regarding home asthma management for a patient with identified barriers to learning.

In this lesson you will learn the essentials of caring for a patient diagnosed with asthma. You will explore the patient's history, evaluate presenting symptoms and treatment upon admission, and follow the patient's progress throughout the hospital stay. Jacqueline Catanazaro is a 45-year-old female admitted with increasing respiratory distress. Begin this lesson by reviewing the general concepts of asthma as presented in your textbook.

Exercise 1

 Clinical Preparation: Writing Activity

⏱ 30 minutes

1. What is another name for asthma?

2. Briefly describe the pathophysiology of asthma.

3. Compare and contrast the four steps of asthma management in the table below.

Steps of Asthma	Clinical Manifestations	Preferred Treatment Recommendations
Step 4 Severe persistent		
Step 3 Moderate persistent		
Step 2 Mild persistent		
Step 1 Mild intermittent		

4. Define the following pulmonary function test measurements. (*Hint:* See Table 61-4 in your textbook.)

    a. Forced vital capacity (FVC)

    b. Forced expiratory volume in the first second (FEV_1)

    c. Peak expiratory flow rate (PEFR)

5. What is a normal PEFR reading? (*Hint:* Look at Figure 61-11 on page 1760 of your textbook.)

Exercise 2

 CD-ROM Activity

 40 minutes

- Sign in to work at Pacific View Regional Hospital for Period of Care 1. (*Note:* If you are already in the virtual hospital from a previous exercise, click on **Leave the Floor** and then **Restart the Program** to get to the sign-in window.)
- From the Patient List, select Jacqueline Catanazaro (Room 402).
- Click on **Go to Nurses' Station**.
- Click on **Chart** and then on **402**.
- Click on **History and Physical**.

1. What medical problems does Jacqueline Catanazaro have?

2. What pathologic triggers can lead to an exacerbation of asthma?

3. Does Jacqueline Catanazaro's history identify any of these triggers?

4. What other factor(s) might be contributing to Jacqueline Catanazaro's asthma exacerbations?

5. Based on Jacqueline Catanazaro's history and home medication regimen, what step of asthma management do you think she is normally at (excluding this admission for an exacerbation)? Explain.

→ • Click on **Emergency Department**.

6. What were Jacqueline Catanazaro's presenting symptoms?

7. What diagnostic testing was ordered? Document and interpret the abnormal results below (*Hint:* Review Laboratory Reports and Diagnostic Reports to obtain these results.)

8. Read the ED physician's progress notes for 1400. What are the results of the patient's PEFR? How would you interpret these in light of her present condition?

→ • Click on **Physician's Orders**.

9. What medical treatment is ordered in the ED? (*Hint:* See orders for Monday at 1005.)

10. How would you evaluate the patient's response to medical treatment?

11. What medications were ordered on Monday at 1600? What is the mechanism of action for each of these drugs? (*Hint:* Return to the Nurses' Station and click on the **Drug Guide** on the counter or on the **Drug** icon in the bottom left corner of your screen.)

12. In what order would the nurse administer these medications? Explain.

13. What new medications are ordered on Tuesday at 0800? Provide a rationale for these orders. Why is the prednisone ordered to be decreased by 5 mg every day?

Exercise 3

 CD-ROM Activity

 30 minutes

- Sign in to work at Pacific View Regional Hospital for Period of Care 1. (*Note:* If you are already in the virtual hospital from a previous exercise, click on **Leave the Floor** and then **Restart the Program** to get to the sign-in window.)
- From the Patient List, select Jacqueline Catanazaro (Room 402).
- Click on **Go to Nurses' Station**.
- Click on **Chart** and then on **402**.
- Click on **Initial Observations**.

1. Describe your initial observations when you enter Jacqueline Catanazaro's room.

- Click on **Take Vital Signs**.

2. Record Jacqueline Catanazaro's vital signs below.

3. Are there any clinical alerts for Jacqueline Catanazaro? If so, describe below.

4. How would you prioritize your care for the patient at this point?

➡ • Click on **Patient Care**.

5. Below, perform and document a focused assessment on three priority areas based on Jacqueline Catanazaro's present status.

Focused Areas of Assessment	Jacqueline's Assessment Findings
a.	
b.	
c.	

➡ • Click on **Chart** and then on **402** for Jacqueline Catanazaro's chart.
• Click on **Physician's Orders**.

6. What new orders did the physician write on Monday at 0730?

➡ • Click on **Return to Room 402**.
• Click on **Nurse-Client Interactions**.
• Select and view the video titled **0730: Intervention—Anxiety**. (*Note:* If this video is not available, check the virtual clock to see whether enough time has elapsed. The video cannot be viewed before its specified time.)

7. How does the nurse in this video prioritize her actions? Give a rationale for these actions?

• Click on **Clinical Alerts**.

   8. Look at the 0800 clinical alert. Interpret this alert below.

 • Click on **Chart** and then on **402**.
  • Click on **Physician's Notes**.

   9. Read the notes for Wednesday at 0800. How does the physician evaluate the patient's condition at this point?

 • Click on **Physician's Orders**.

  10. Below, record the orders for 0800 on Wednesday. Provide a rationale or expected therapeutic response for each order.

New Orders   **Rationale/Expected Therapeutic Response**

Exercise 4

 CD-ROM Activity

 45 minutes

- Sign in to work at Pacific View Regional Hospital for Period of Care 2. (*Note:* If you are already in the virtual hospital from a previous exercise, click on **Leave the Floor** and then **Restart the Program** to get to the sign-in window.)
- From the Patient List, select Jacqueline Catanazaro (Room 402).
- Click on **Get Report**.

1. Briefly summarize the activity for Jacqueline Catanazaro over the last 4 hours.

- Click on **Go to Nurses' Station**.
- Click on **402** to go to the patient's room.

2. What is your initial observation of Jacqueline Catanazaro for this time period?

3. Are there any clinical alerts?

- Click on **Take Vital Signs**.

4. Record the patient's vital signs below. How do these results compare with those you obtained during Period of Care 1? (*Hint:* See Exercise 3, question 2 of this lesson.)

- Click on **Patient Care**.

5. Perform a focused assessment on Jacqueline Catanazaro and record your findings in the middle column below. In the last column, compare these findings with those you obtained during Period of Care 1. Interpret your results. (*Hint:* See Exercise 3, question 5.)

Focused Areas of Assessment	Current Findings	Comparison with 0800 Findings— Interpretation of Results
Respiratory		
Cardiovascular		
Mental Status		

 • Click on **Nurse-Client Interactions**.
- Select and view the video titled **1115: Assessment—Readiness to Learn**. (*Note:* If this video is not available, check the virtual clock to see whether enough time has elapsed. The video cannot be viewed before its specified time.)

6. Describe the nurse's actions in the video. Are they appropriate? Explain.

7. What barriers to learning might be present for Jacqueline Catanazaro?

- Click on **Leave the Floor**.
- Click on **Restart the Program**.
- Sign in for Period of Care 3.
- From the Patient List, select Jacqueline Catanazaro (Room 402).
- Click on **Go to Nurses' Station** and then on **402** to return to the patient's room.
- Click on **Patient Care**.
- Click on **Nurse-Client Interactions**.
- Select and view the video titled **1500: Intervention—Patient Teaching**. (*Note:* If this video is not available, check the virtual clock to see whether enough time has elapsed. The video cannot be viewed before its specified time.)

8. In the video, what equipment is the nurse teaching the patient about?

9. Describe the proper use of the peak flow meter for this patient. (*Hint:* See Client Education Guide on page 1816 of your textbook.)

10. What should Jacqueline Catanazaro be taught regarding the results of her peak flow measurements?

11. Describe the directions you would give Jacqueline Catanazaro for properly using a metered-dose inhaler (MDI).

12. What other asthma management needs would you teach the patient?

→ • Click on **Chart** and then on **402** for Jacqueline Catanazaro's record.
   • Click on **Patient Education**.

13. What are the educational goals for Jacqueline Catanazaro?

14. Describe the differences in outcomes met for the patient and her sister.

15. The patient is scheduled for discharge tomorrow. Do you have any concerns? What would be your most appropriate action?

DVT/Pulmonary Embolism

Reading Assignment: Management of Clients with Vascular Disorders (Chapter 55)
Management of Clients with Lower Airway and
Pulmonary Vessel Disorders (Chapter 63)

Patient: Clarence Hughes, Room 404

Goal: Utilize the nursing process to competently care for patients with a critically altered oxygenation state.

Objectives:

1. Identify clinical manifestations of pulmonary embolism.
2. Prioritize nursing care for a patient with acute onset of respiratory distress and chest pain.
3. Describe diagnostic testing relative to the diagnosis of pulmonary embolism.
4. Describe pharmacologic therapy for patient with pulmonary embolism.
5. Accurately calculate correct dosage of heparin for patient using a sliding scale.
6. Identify disease management issues regarding the care of a patient with pulmonary embolism.

In this lesson you will learn the essentials of caring for a patient diagnosed with an acute pulmonary embolism as a sequela of deep vein thrombosis. You will explore the patient's history, evaluate presenting symptoms and treatment, provide appropriate nursing interventions, and assess the patient's progress throughout the clinical day. Clarence Hughes is a 73-year-old male admitted for an elective left knee arthroplasty.

Exercise 1

 CD-ROM Activity

 30 minutes

- Sign in to work at Pacific View Regional Hospital for Period of Care 2. (*Note:* If you are already in the virtual hospital from a previous exercise, click on **Leave the Floor** and then **Restart the Program** to get to the sign-in window.)
- From the Patient List, select Clarence Hughes (Room 404).
- Click on **Get Report**.

1. Before entering Clarence Hughes' room, summarize what you would expect to find based on the report you received.

→ • Click on **Go to Nurses' Station**.
 • Click on **404** to go to Clarence Hughes' room.

2. What is your initial observation as you enter the patient's room?

3. What should your priority actions be at this point?

→ • Click on **Patient Care**.
 • Click on **Nurse-Client Interactions**.
 • Select and view the video titled **1115: Interventions—Airway**. (*Note:* If this video is not available, check the virtual clock to see whether enough time has elapsed. The video cannot be viewed before its specified time.)

4. Describe the nurse's actions in this video. Should the nurse have left the patient to go get oxygen? Explain your answer. If not, what else could she have done?

5. What signs or symptoms of pulmonary embolus is Clarence Hughes displaying?

6. Suspecting a pulmonary embolus, what other clinical manifestations would you assess Clarence Hughes for?

➤ • Click on **Chart** and then on **404** for Clarence Hughes' record.
   • Click on **History and Physical**.

7. Based on the patient's history and current reason for hospitalization, what risk factors for DVT and resultant pulmonary embolus does Clarence Hughes have?

➤ • Click on **Physician's Orders**.

8. Look at the orders dated Wednesday at 1120. Document these orders below and provide a rationale for each.

Physician Order	**Rationale**

• Click on **Return to Room 404**.
- Click on **Patient Care** and then on **Nurse-Client Interactions**.
- Select and view the video titled **1135: Change in Patient Condition**.

9. As the nurse in the video explains care to the family, she states that a transporter will be coming to take Clarence Hughes for a ventilation-perfusion scan. Would you send this patient down to radiology with just the transporter? Why or why not?

Exercise 2

 CD-ROM Activity

 30 minutes

- Sign in to work at Pacific View Regional Hospital for Period of Care 3. (*Note:* If you are already in the virtual hospital from a previous exercise, click on **Leave the Floor** and then **Restart the Program** to get to the sign-in window.)
- From the Patient List, select Clarence Hughes (Room 404).
- Click on **Go to Nurses' Station**.
- Click on **Chart** and then on **404**.
- Click on **Laboratory Reports** and **Diagnostic Reports**.

1. Document the results of the ordered diagnostic testing below.

Diagnostic Test	Result

• Click on **Physician's Orders**.

   2. What orders were written to treat Clarence Hughes' pulmonary embolus?

   3. What lab test will be used to titrate the heparin infusion?

   4. What is the desired therapeutic level for this lab test? (*Hint:* You may consult the Drug Guide in the Nurses' Station.)

 • Click on **Return to Nurses' Station**.
   • Click on **MAR** and then on **404** for Clarence Hughes' record.

   5. How many mL of heparin would you administer for the bolus dose?

   6. If you were the nurse starting the heparin infusion, at what rate would you set the IV pump to infuse this medication?

 • Click on **Return to Nurses' Station**.
   • Click on **Chart** and then on **404** for Clarence Hughes' record.
   • Click on **Laboratory Reports**.

   7. What were the results of the aPTT and INR at 1300 today? Why were these tests ordered prior to starting the heparin?

• Click on **Return to Nurses' Station**.
• Click on **404** to enter Clarence Hughes' room.
• Click on **Patient Care** and then on **Patient-Client Interactions**.
• Select and view the video titled **1510: Disease Management**. (*Note:* If this video is not available, check the virtual clock to see whether enough time has elapsed. The video cannot be viewed before its specified time.)

8. When the son asks the nurse whether the pulmonary embolism will delay his father's discharge, the nurse states that the heparin takes 2 days to stabilize. Does this mean that the patient will be discharged on heparin? If not, what medication will be used to minimize clot formation? Explain why the patient is not started on this medication rather than heparin.

9. What lab test(s) will be used to monitor the therapeutic effect of Coumadin? What is the therapeutic range for these tests?

10. For what possible complications would you monitor Clarence Hughes related to the pulmonary embolism?

Exercise 3

 CD-ROM Activity

 30 minutes

• Sign in to work at Pacific View Regional Hospital for Period of Care 4. (*Note:* If you are already in the virtual hospital from a previous exercise, click on **Leave the Floor** and then **Restart the Program** to get to the sign-in window.)
• From the Patient List, select Clarence Hughes (Room 404).
• Click on **Go to Nurses' Station**.
• Click on **Chart** and then on **404**.
• Click on **Laboratory Reports**.

1. What is the aPTT result for 1900?

➤ • Click on **Return to Nurses' Station**.
 • Click on **MAR** and then on **404** for Clarence Hughes' record.

2. What would you do now with the heparin infusion? Calculate the correct infusion rate below. (*Hint:* Refer to your answer for question 7 in Exercise 2.)

➤ • Click on **Return to Nurses' Station**.
 • Click on **Kardex** and then on **404** for Clarence Hughes' record.

3. Are there any other outcomes that should be added based on the patient's current set-back? Explain.

4. If the heparin is not effective in treating Clarence Hughes and/or his condition worsens, what other pharmacologic treatment might be helpful? Explain.

5. Describe bleeding precautions that must be followed while Clarence Hughes is receiving heparin therapy.

6. If Clarence Hughes' condition deteriorates, what surgical treatment might be needed? Explain.

7. If Clarence Hughes develops another pulmonary embolus while being treated with anticoagulation, what additional treatment might the physician consider to prevent the recurrence of PE? Explain.

Emphysema and Pneumonia

 Reading Assignment: Management of Clients with Lower Airway and
Pulmonary Vessel Disorders (Chapter 63)
Management of Clients with Parenchymal and
Pleural Disorders (Chapter 64)

Patient: Patricia Newman, Room 406

Goal: Utilize the nursing process to competently care for patients with altered oxygenation
states.

Objectives:

1. Relate physical assessment findings with pathophysiologic changes of the lower respiratory
   tract.
2. Prioritize nursing care for a patient with altered oxygenation.
3. Evaluate laboratory results relative to the diagnosis of pneumonia and emphysema.
4. Describe pharmacologic interventions related to altered oxygenation states.
5. Identify appropriate nursing interventions for a patient admitted with pneumonia and
   emphysema.
6. Identify appropriate discharge teaching needs for a patient with altered oxygenation.

In this lesson you will learn the essentials of caring for a patient diagnosed with pneumonia and
emphysema. You will explore the patient's history, evaluate presenting symptoms and treatment
upon admission, and assess the patient's progress throughout the hospital stay. Patricia Newman
is a 61-year-old female admitted with pneumonia and a history of emphysema. Begin this lesson
by reviewing the general concepts of altered oxygenation states as presented in your textbook.

Exercise 1

 Clinical Preparation: Writing Activity

20 minutes

1. What category(ies) of lung diseases does emphysema belong to?

2. Briefly describe the pathophysiology of emphysema.

3. Briefly describe the pathophysiology of pneumonia.

4. What are the major risk factors for pneumonia?

Exercise 2

 CD-ROM Activity

 45 minutes

- Sign in to work at Pacific View Regional Hospital for Period of Care 1. (*Note:* If you are already in the virtual hospital from a previous exercise, click on **Leave the Floor** and then **Restart the Program** to get to the sign-in window.)
- From the Patient List, select Patricia Newman (Room 406).
- Click on **Get Report**.

1. What questions would you ask the outgoing nurses to obtain needed information not identified in report?

2. Below, relate the clinical manifestations identified in the change-of-shift report to the patient's diagnosis of pneumonia.

Clinical Manifestations	Pathophysiologic Basis
Labored respirations	
Use of accessory muscles	
Productive cough with yellow sputum	
Course breath sounds	
Lung infiltrates	
Disturbed sleep patterns	
Tachycardia	
Fever	

→ • Click on **Go to Nurses' Station**.
  • Click on **Chart** and then on **406** for Patricia Newman's chart.
  • Click on **History and Physical**.

3. What risk factors for pneumonia does Patricia Newman have?

→ • Click on **Nursing Admission**.

4. What other risk factor for pneumonia is documented on the Nursing Admission form? (*Hint:* Look for something that might have prevented the pneumonia.)

→ • Click on **Return to Nurses' Station**.
  • Click on **406** to enter Patricia Newman's room.
  • Click on **Initial Observation**.

5. What would be your priority nursing assessment/intervention(s) based on this initial observation?

→ • Click on **Patient Care**.

6. Perform a focused clinical assessment based on Patricia Newman's admitting diagnosis and record your findings below. How has Patricia Newman's condition changed since report?

Focused Assessment Area	Assessment Findings	Change in Assessment

 • Click on **Nurse-Client Interactions**.
   • Select and view the video titled **0730: Prioritizing Interventions**. (*Note:* If this video is not available, check the virtual clock to see whether enough time has elapsed. The video cannot be viewed before its specified time.)

7. Evaluate the nurse's actions based on the patient's current status. How does this nurse's action differ from your plan of care as answered in question 5?

8. What nursing interventions might alleviate Patricia Newman's anxiety and improve her activity tolerance?

➤ • Click on **Chart** and then on **406** for Patricia Newman's record.
   • Click on **Laboratory Reports**.

9. Identify any abnormal lab results and describe how they correlate with Patricia Newman's diagnosis of pneumonia.

➤ • Click on **Return to Room 406**.
   • Click on **MAR** and select tab **406**.

10. What is the desired therapeutic effect of ipatroprium bromide? How could the nurse assess whether the desired effect was achieved?

11. What is the desired therapeutic effect of cefotetan? How could the nurse assess whether the desired effect was achieved?

12. What is the rationale for administration of IV fluids related to pneumonia?

Medication Preparation

 • Click on **Medication Room**.

• Click on **MAR** to determine medications that Patricia Newman is ordered to receive at 0800 and any appropriate prn medications you may want to administer. (*Note:* You may click on **Review MAR** at any time to verify correct medication order. Remember to look at the patient name on the MAR to make sure you have the correct patient's record—you must click on the correct room number within the MAR.) Click on **Return to Medication Room** after reviewing the MAR.

• Click on **Unit Dosage**. When the close-up view appears, click on drawer **406**.

• Select the medication(s) you plan to administer. After each medication you select, click **Put Medication on Tray**. When you are finished, click on **Close Drawer**.

• Click **View Medication Room**.

• Click on **IV Storage**. From the close-up view, click on the drawer labeled **Large Volume**.

• Select the medication(s) you plan to administer, put medication(s) on tray, and close bin.

• Click **View Medication Room**.

• Click on **Preparation**. Select the correct medication to administer; click **Prepare** and **Next.**

• Choose the correct patient to administer this medication to and click **Finish**.

• Repeat the above two steps until all medications that you want to administer are prepared.

• You can click **Review Your Medications** and then **Return to Medication Room** when ready. From the Medication Room, you may go directly to Patricia Newman's room by clicking on **406** at bottom of screen.

Medication Administration

 • Administer the medication, utilizing the five rights of medication administration. After you have collected the appropriate assessment data and are ready for administration, click **Patient Care** and then **Medication Administration**. Verify that the correct patient and medication(s) appear in the left-hand window. Then click the down arrow next to Select. From the drop-down menu, select **Administer** and complete the Administration Wizard by providing any information requested. When the Wizard stops asking for information, click **Administer to Patient**. Specify **Yes** when asked whether this administration should be recorded in the MAR. Finally, click **Finish**.

Now let's see how you did!

 • Click on **Leave the Floor** at the bottom of your screen. From the Floor Menu, select **Look at Your Preceptor's Evaluation**. Then click on **Medication Scorecard**.

13. Note below whether or not you correctly administered the appropriate medications. If not, why do you think you were incorrect? According to Table C in this scorecard, what are the appropriate resources that should be used and important assessments that should be completed before administering these medications? Did you use these resources and perform these assessments correctly?

Exercise 3

 CD-ROM Activity

 40 minutes

- Sign in to work at Pacific View Regional Hospital for Period of Care 2. (*Note:* If you are already in the virtual hospital from a previous exercise, click on **Leave the Floor** and then **Restart the Program** to get to the sign-in window.)
- From the Patient List, select Patricia Newman (Room 406).
- Click on **Go to Nurses' Station**.
- Click on **Chart** and then on **406** for Patricia Newman's record.
- Click on **History and Physical**.

1. How long has Patricia Newman been diagnosed with emphysema?

2. What clinical manifestations documented on the H&P can be attributed to emphysema?

3. What additional clinical manifestations might you expect to see in other patients with emphysema?

- Click on **Diagnostic Reports**.

4. What findings on the CXR are consistent with the diagnosis of emphysema?

5. What is the relationship between the patient's admitting diagnosis (pneumonia) and her underlying chronic condition (emphysema)?

6. What other pulmonary complication of emphysema should the nurse be alert for in Patricia Newman? Explain the pathophysiologic basis for this occurrence.

➡ • Click on **Physician's Orders**.

7. What is the order for oxygen?

8. What is the rationale for this oxygen order as opposed to the usual goal of greater than 90%-93% oxygen saturation?

➡ • Click on **Patient Education**.

9. What is educational goal 3 for Patricia Newman?

10. Explain the rationale for using this breathing technique.

11. What is educational goal 4 for Patricia Newman?

12. What do you think Patricia Newman's special dietary needs are? Explain your answer.

 13. Since Patricia Newman's emphysema puts her at high risk for pulmonary infections, what would you teach her to do to help prevent further episodes of pneumonia? (*Hint:* See NCP on page 1828 of the textbook.)

 • Click on **Return to Nurses' Station** and then on **406** to go to Patricia Newman's room.
   • Inside the room, click on **Patient Care** and then on **Nurse-Client Interactions**.
   • Select and view the video titled **1100: Care Coordination**. (*Note:* If this video is not available, check the virtual clock to see whether enough time has elapsed. The video cannot be viewed before its specified time.)

14. What disciplines are involved in planning and providing care for Patricia Newman? Explain the role of each person in helping meet the patient's health care needs by completing the chart below.

Involved Disciplines	Role in Patricia's Health Care

LESSON **23** —————————————————

Glaucoma

 Reading Assignment: Management of Clients with Visual Disorders (Chapter 67)

Patient: Clarence Hughes, Room 404

Goal: Utilize the nursing process to competently care for patients with glaucoma.

Objectives:

1. Describe the pathophysiology of glaucoma.
2. Identify clinical manifestations related to glaucoma.
3. Describe appropriate pharmacologic treatment of glaucoma.
4. Administer eye drops safely and accurately.
5. Evaluate a patient's ability to correctly administered prescribed ophthalmic medication.

In this lesson you will learn the essentials of caring for a patient diagnosed with glaucoma. You will explore the patient's history, evaluate presenting symptoms and treatment, administer prescribed medications, and develop an individualized discharge teaching plan. Clarence Hughes is a 73-year-old male admitted for an elective left knee arthroplasty.

Exercise 1

 Clinical Preparation: Writing Activity

15 minutes

1. Describe the pathophysiology of glaucoma.

2. Identify and describe the two major types of glaucoma.

   a.

   b.

3. Identify factors associated with the development of open-angle glaucoma.

Exercise 2

 CD-ROM Activity

 45 minutes

- Sign in to work at Pacific View Regional Hospital for Period of Care 3. (*Note:* If you are already in the virtual hospital from a previous exercise, click on **Leave the Floor** and then **Restart the Program** to get to the sign-in window.)
- From the Patient List, select Clarence Hughes (Room 404).
- Click on **Go to Nurses' Station**.
- Click on **Chart** and then on **404** for Clarence Hughes' record.
- Click on **History and Physical**.

1. What problems of the eye does Clarence Hughes have?

 2. How would this be diagnosed? (*Hint:* See pages 1927-1928 of your textbook.)

3. What signs and symptoms do you think Clarence Hughes had prior to diagnosis?

4. For what clinical manifestation(s) and/or history should you assess Clarence Hughes related to this diagnosis?

5. The History and Physical does not identify the type of glaucoma Clarence Hughes has. Based on his history and the information in your textbook, which type do you think he mostly likely has? Explain why you came to this conclusion.

 • Click on **Return to Nurses' Station**.
 • Click on **MAR** and then on **404** for Clarence Hughes' record.

6. What medications are ordered for Clarence Hughes' glaucoma? Identify these medications, their classifications, and mechanisms of action below. You will complete the last column in question 7. (*Hint:* You may consult the Drug Guide in the Nurses' Station.)

Medication	Drug Classification	Mechanism of Action	Side Effects

7. For what side effects should you monitor Clarence Hughes related to these medications? Record your answer in the table after question 6.

8. If you were to administer the prescribed antiglaucoma medication to Clarence Hughes, how would you correctly apply the eye drops? Explain the step-by-step procedure.

9. What would you expect Clarence Hughes' tonometry reading to be during treatment of his glaucoma?

10. Identify an appropriate outcome for Clarence Hughes related to his glaucoma.

→ • Click on **Return to Nurses' Station**.
 • Click on **Chart** and then on **404** for Clarence Hughes' record.
 • Click on **Patient Education**.

11. What educational goals would you add for Clarence Hughes related to his glaucoma?

12. What teaching would you provide Clarence Hughes regarding his glaucoma?

13. Complete the following table by documenting the teaching points you would you review with Clarence Hughes regarding his glaucoma medications.

Medication	Teaching Points

14. What teaching methods would you use to teach medication administration?

15. How would you evaluate Clarence Hughes' understanding of correct application?

16. If Clarence Hughes' ophthalmic medications fail to maintain his IOP within normal limits, what other therapy might he expect to undergo? Briefly explain these procedures.

LESSON **24**

Low Back Pain

 Reading Assignment: Management of Clients with Peripheral Nervous System Disorders (Chapter 73)

Patient: Jacqueline Catanazaro, Room 402

Goal: Utilize the nursing process to competently care for patients with an intervertebral disc problem.

Objectives:

1. Describe the pathophysiology of low back pain.
2. Identify clinical manifestations related to low back pain and/or herniated intervertebral disc.
3. Plan appropriate interventions to treat low back pain.
4. Evaluate a patient's potential to comply with a health care management plan.
5. Develop an individualized teaching plan for a patient with low back pain.

In this lesson you will learn the essentials of caring for a patient experiencing chronic low back pain. You will explore the patient's history, evaluate presenting symptoms and treatment, plan appropriate nursing interventions to treat the patient's symptoms, and develop an individualized discharge teaching plan. Jacqueline Catanazaro is a 45-year-old female admitted with an acute exacerbation of asthma.

Exercise 1

 Clinical Preparation: Writing Activity

10 minutes

1. Describe the underlying pathophysiology of low back pain.

2. Define the following procedures.

   a. Percutaneous diskectomy

   b. Microdiskectomy

   c. Decompressive laminectomy

   d. Artificial disk replacement

   e. Spinal fusion (arthodesis)

Exercise 2

 CD-ROM Activity

 45 minutes

- Sign in to work at Pacific View Regional Hospital for Period of Care 3. (*Note:* If you are already in the virtual hospital from a previous exercise, click on **Leave the Floor** and then **Restart the Program** to get to the sign-in window.)
- From the Patient List, select Jacqueline Catanazaro (Room 402).
- Click on **Go to Nurses' Station**.
- Click on **Chart** and then on **402** for Jacqueline Catanazaro's record.
- Click on **History and Physical**.

1. Under "History of Present Illness," what are Jacqueline Catanazaro's complaints related to her back?

2. How does the physician describe this problem under "Past Medical History"?

3. How was this diagnosed?

4. How long has she had this problem?

5. What treatment has she undergone? Explain the mechanism of action and/or rationale for these treatments.

6. What assessment should be completed on Jacqueline Catanazaro in relation to the back pain?

→ • Click on **Nurse's Notes**.

7. How have the nurses addressed Jacqueline Catanazaro's complaints of low back pain?

8. What interventions can you suggest that would be appropriate to control Jacqueline Catanazaro's pain?

 • Click on **History and Physical**.

 9. What is the physician's plan regarding this patient's back pain? What type of interventions might be offered by this intervention? (*Hint:* See Chapter 22 of your textbook.)

10. What interventions would you plan to improve Jacqueline Catanazaro's mobility and thus her activity level?

11. If Jacqueline Catanazaro's back pain persists with the current medical management, does research support the use of surgical therapy to improve her clinical outcome?

12. If Jacqueline Catanazaro would decide to undergo surgery in an effort to find pain relief, for what potential postoperative problems/complications would you need to monitor her?

→ • Click on **Patient Education**.

13. What goals related to Jacqueline Catanazaro's back pain would you add?

→ • Click on **History and Physical**.

14. What may interfere with Jacqueline Catanazaro's compliance to health care instructions?

• Click on **Return to Nurses' Station**.
• Click on **402** to enter Jacqueline Catanazaro's room.
• Inside her room, click on **Patient Care** and then on **Nurse-Client Interactions**.
• Select and view the video titled **1540: Discharge Planning**. (*Note:* If this video is not available, check the virtual clock to see whether enough time has elapsed. The video cannot be viewed before its specified time.)

 15. After viewing the video, what other suggestions do you have for assisting Jacqueline Catanazaro with compliance after discharge? (*Hint:* See Chapter 1 in your textbook.)

LESSON **25** —————————————————————————

Transfusion Therapy

 Reading Assignment: Management of Clients with Hematologic Disorders
(Chapter 77)

Patient: Piya Jordan, Room 403

Goal: Utilize the nursing process to competently care for patients receiving various blood
products.

Objectives:

1. Describe the ABO and Rh antigen systems.
2. Identify the correct type blood to administer to a specific patient.
3. Describe appropriate nursing responsibilities related to blood product administration.
4. Evaluate vital sign assessments related to potential blood transfusion reactions.
5. Describe appropriate assessment parameters when monitoring for various types of transfusion reactions.

In this lesson you will learn the essentials of caring for a patient receiving blood and blood
product transfusions. You will describe pretransfusion responsibilities, identify administration
specifics, and evaluate the patient during and after each transfusion. Piya Jordan is a 68-year-old
female admitted with nausea, vomiting, and abdominal pain.

Exercise 1

 Clinical Preparation: Writing Activity

10 minutes

1. Describe the ABO antigen system. (*Hint:* Read page 2253 of your textbook.)

2. Describe the Rh antigen system.

 3. Complete the following table to identify which types of blood are compatible with each other. (*Hint:* Use Table 77-3 in your textbook.)

Patient's Blood Type	Blood Types That This Patient May Receive
A+	
A–	
B+	
B–	
O+	
O–	
AB+	
AB–	

Exercise 2

 CD-ROM Activity

 30 minutes

- Sign in to work at Pacific View Regional Hospital for Period of Care 1. (*Note:* If you are already in the virtual hospital from a previous exercise, click on **Leave the Floor** and then **Restart the Program** to get to the sign-in window.)
- From the Patient List, select Piya Jordan (Room 403).
- Click on **Go to Nurses' Station**.
- Click on **Chart** and then on **403** to access Piya Jordan's records.
- Click on **Laboratory Reports**.

1. Record Piya Jordan's hematology results below.

	Monday 2200	Tuesday 0630	Wednesday 0630
Hemoglobin			
Hematocrit			

2. Why do you think Piya Jordan's H&H is lower on Wednesday? (*Hint:* Check the Physican's Notes in the chart.)

 • Click on **Physician's Orders**.

3. What was ordered to correct this? Is this appropriate related to Piya Jordan's level of hemo-globin? Explain why or why not.

 • Click on **Return to Nurses' Station** and then on **403** to enter Piya Jordan's room.
   • Inside her room, click on **Patient Care** and then on **Nurse-Client Interactions**.
   • Select and view the video titled **0735: Pain—Adverse Drug Event**. (*Note:* If this video is not available, check the virtual clock to see whether enough time has elapsed. The video cannot be viewed before its specified time.)

4. What does the nurse state she will do to prepare Piya Jordan for a blood transfusion?

5. What gauge IV would you insert for the blood transfusion?

- Click on **Chart** and then on **403** for Piya Jordan's records.
- Click on **Laboratory Reports**.

6. What pretransfusion testing must be completed? Are these documented on Piya Jordan's chart?

7. What other pretransfusion responsibilities would you complete prior to requesting blood release?

8. Explain how you would prepare the blood set-up prior to administration? What types of solutions can and cannot be infused with blood products?

Exercise 3

 CD-ROM Activity

 30 minutes

- Sign in to work at Pacific View Regional Hospital for Period of Care 2. (*Note:* If you are already in the virtual hospital from a previous exercise, click on **Leave the Floor** and then **Restart the Program** to get to the sign-in window.)
- From the Patient List, select Piya Jordan (Room 403).
- Click on **403** to enter Piya Jordan's room.
- Click on **Patient Care**.
- Click on **Nurse-Client Interactions**.
- Select and view the video titled **1115: Interventions—Nausea and Blood**. (*Note:* If this video is not available, check the virtual clock to see whether enough time has elapsed. The video cannot be viewed before its specified time.)

1. Piya Jordan's daughter voices concern regarding the safety of blood transfusion. How did the nurse respond to this?

2. Describe how you would explain the safety of blood transfusions.

3. During the video, the nurse states that the blood has just arrived. How soon should the nurse begin the transfusion?

➤ • Click on **Chart** and then on **403**.
  • Click on **Laboratory Reports**.

4. What is Piya Jordan's blood type?

5. What type of blood may she receive safely?

6. Describe the nurse's responsibilities during the initiation of this transfusion.

7. What assessments should be completed on Piya Jordan during the transfusion?

8. What would you do if Piya Jordan displayed any unusual manifestations during the blood transfusion?

9. What would you document regarding this blood transfusion?

Exercise 4

 CD-ROM Activity

 40 minutes

- Sign in to work at Pacific View Regional Hospital for Period of Care 4. (*Note:* If you are already in the virtual hospital from a previous exercise, click on **Leave the Floor** and then **Restart the Program** to get to the sign-in window.)
- From the Patient List, select Piya Jordan (Room 403).
- Click on **Go to Nurses' Station**.
- Click on **EPR** and **Login**.
- Select **403** as the patient's room number and **Vital Signs** as the category.

1. Below, document Piya Jordan's vital signs as recorded in the EPR after each of the two units of blood.

	1130	1145	1200	1250	1315	1400
Temp						
Pulse						
BP						
Resp						

	1415	1430	1445	1500	1515	1530
Temp						
Pulse						
BP						
Resp						

2. According to the vital sign findings above, did Piya Jordan have any adverse reaction(s) to the blood transfusions? Explain.

3. What type of symptoms might be present if Piya Jordan had a hemolytic transfusion reaction?

4. How would these symptoms differ if Piya Jordan would have an allergic transfusion reaction?

5. How can you determine that Piya Jordan did not have a febrile reaction if she was febrile at the beginning of the transfusion?

6. What was Piya Jordan's total intake and output over the last 24 hours (Tuesday at 1500 through Wednesday at 1500)?

→ • Click on **Exit EPR**.
 • Click on **MAR** and then on **403** for Piya Jordan's records.

7. Over what period of time was the first unit of RBC infused? Was this appropriate? Explain.

8. What signs or symptoms would you expect to see if Piya Jordan was suffering from circulatory overload?

→ • Click on **Return to Nurses' Station**.
 • Click on **Chart** and then on **403** to access Piya Jordan's records.
 • Click on **Expired MARs**.

9. What other blood product has Piya Jordan received this admission? (*Hint:* Check Tuesday's MAR.)

10. How does the product you identified in question 9 differ from RBCs? Why was it given to Piya Jordan? (*Hint:* Check the History and Physical to determine the reason for giving it to Piya Jordan.)

11. How does administration of FFP differ from administration of RBCs?

Notes:

Notes:

Notes:

Notes: